" For tens of millions of patients, Covid continues to cause lingering effects that compromise their quality of life. Many will find the straightforward and practical information in *The Covid Long Haul Solution* to be an immensely helpful companion as they navigate this uncertain path."

—Robert M. Wachter, MD, Professor and Chair,
Department of Medicine, University of California,
author of *The New York Times* bestseller, *The Digital Doctor*

" An invaluable resource for those seeking a return to normalcy. In *The Long COVID Solution,* Dr. Kuon provides a comprehensive holistic regimen that will surely help many regain their health, or even improve it!"

—Donald I. Abrams, MD, Integrative Oncology,
UCSF Osher Center for Integrative Health,
Professor Emeritus of Medicine,
University of California San Francisco

THE
LONG COVID
SOLUTION

A holistic integrative approach to post-viral recovery

CARLA KUON, MD

Pia Publishing
CARLAKUONMD.COM

Interior design and editing: John Byrne Barry
Cover design: Ruth Schwartz
Cover Photo: Shutterstock Stock Images

Publisher's Catalog data
Names: Kuon, Carla, author

Title: The Long COVID Solution
ISBN: 979-8-9875655-1-0
Library of Congress Control Number: 2023901479

Subjects: Long COVID|Post-viral recovery|Chronic Fatigue Syndrome | Myalgic Encephalitis

Contents

PREFACE

How To Use This Book

When I started writing this book, I intended to craft a simple guide on how to choose the best diet and supplements to resolve symptoms associated with Long COVID. However, once I started writing the manuscript, it became clear that it was important to explain not only the *how* of using the protocol, but to explain the *why* as well. One of my goals as an integrative physician is to help patients by obtaining diagnostics to inform targeted and personalized treatment recommendations. Another equally important goal is to educate patients. Knowledge empowers them to better manage their symptoms. In my specialty of integrative medicine, this is accomplished largely through natural interventions and lifestyle changes. I spend an hour with each patient and thus I have the time to explain the *how* as well as the *why*. The knowledge gained increases patient independence and helps them to regain a sense of control over health outcomes, often resulting in decreased utilization of strained medical resources. With knowledge and empowerment, patients are better able to advocate for themselves while navigating an increasingly complex medical system.

Chronic fatigue syndrome (CFS) is a devastating condition which has largely been ignored by the medical community and is treated by only a handful of clinicians across the country. Most patients and clinicians are often at a loss on how to approach chronic fatigue. Many of these patients find their way to integrative care providers. Clinicians trained in integrative medicine are therefore well positioned to treat Long COVID because of striking similarities with CFS. As such, this book evolved to be both a guide and a teaching tool. I have included the science behind my recommendations so that both patients and those caring for COVID survivors can have a better sense on how to manage their perplexing constellation of symptoms. This book is not comprehensive of all potential pathways activated by COVID nor all the organs which can be affected by COVID, but the most common inflammatory pathways which are of highest yield. For example, I do not specifically address myocarditis, a well-known complication of COVID that is less frequent than neuroinflammation, brain fog, and exercise intolerance. Instead, I address the underlying inflammation, which can affect all organs, including the heart.

My goal in this book is twofold: to present a holistic protocol for Long COVID, and to explain the underlying biology of Long COVID, hoping to increase awareness in the general community about diagnostic and treatment options. The clinician who reads this book will hopefully emerge with a better understanding of how to treat Long COVID and CFS, given their similarities. The patient who reads this book will hopefully understand how to improve their symptoms at home and how to better advocate for themselves in the medical community.

I have structured each chapter to contain explanations of the science behind each recommendation, and the recommendations summarized separately at the end. If you are experiencing brain fog from Long COVID, the science may prove too much of a cognitive load. You are welcome to skip to the friendly summarized bullet points in each chapter. Those with brain fatigue can concentrate their energy on reading the chapter on the anti-inflammatory diet, and the summarized supplement recommendations at the end of chapter 7. As you improve, you may wish to read the explanations in each chapter to understand the *why*. If you are science-driven and would like to understand the physiology of Long COVID and the evidence behind my recommendations, I have provided references from the clinical trials and peer-reviewed publications that have informed this protocol.

In my career as an integrative medicine physician, I have been amazed at the power of proper nutrition, when combined with carefully selected supplements. My initial curiosity about the power of plants began when I was an attending physician in the bone marrow transplant service at the University of California, San Francisco (UCSF). During my seven years as a hospitalist there I learned of several life-saving cancer drugs that came from plants: mustard seeds gave us a therapy called cyclophosphamide, the periwinkle flower gave us vinca alkaloids such as vincristine and vinblastine. A regimen with high dose vitamin A was the basis for a protocol called ATRAA, which revolutionized the treatment of promyelocytic leukemia—turning this once deadly cancer into a highly treatable one with astounding success. Those years deepened my understanding of immunology and my curiosity about natural remedies. A question was planted in my brain that I couldn't ignore: what if we used our knowledge of the chemicals found in plants to prevent serious disease or turn around chronic illness? Once this seed planted itself in my brain, I couldn't shake it. It led me to pursue a fellowship at UCSF's Osher Center for Integrative Health, where I have been faculty ever since. Learning plant medicines felt like going to medical school all over again—the vast pharmacopeia of plants is complicated by plants having many chemicals, not just one, increasing the complexity of choice. However, once I started applying my knowledge of plants to my understanding of human physiology, the improvements promoted in health and well-being have repeatedly astounded me.

Conventional medicine takes a catastrophic "don't fix it if it isn't broken" approach, while integrative medicine seeks to optimize health in everybody by identifying and correcting the underlying drivers of illness. Each has merits in health care. Broken bones and acute life-threatening illness are best treated by conventional methods when time is of the essence. Conditions that lead to chronic illness often benefit from a holistic approach, as chronic illness has multiple drivers contributing to the symptoms. There are two competing axioms of diagnosis in medicine: Occam's Razor, a philosophy in which the single best diagnosis that explains all the symptoms must be the correct one. In chronic illness, this oversimplification yields poor outcomes for the patient. In this scenario, every fatigued patient gets labeled with fibromyalgia, and there is nothing else to do for them. Hickam's Dictum, on the other hand, tells us "A patient can have as many diseases as they damn well please." Hickam's Dictum encourages the clinician to investigate all the factors in the case, and is more appropriate for chronic illness, since human biology is enormously complex.

Any clinician who treats CFS knows that conventional medicine has limited and often unsatisfactory treatment options, and this clinician must avail themselves of every recourse to help relieve the suffering of their patients. Most integrative physicians therefore treat chronic fatigue by using both drugs and natural remedies, and by early adoption of advanced diagnostic tools such as human microbiome testing. Integrative medicine physicians therefore push the envelope of conventional medicine's comfort by combining natural interventions with conventional approaches. This tension can elicit pushback from conventional medicine, even disapproval. Yet in a world with a rising prevalence of chronic illness, and in the post COVID era in particular, patients increasingly demand this dual approach. They want doctors who have one foot in each world—who can diagnose and treat rare disease, but who can also teach them natural approaches to managing their health. At a minimum, they expect a health care team that can collaborate with integrative methods, not discourage them.

As an academically trained, double board-certified physician—a doctor with one foot in each world—I am committed to practicing evidence-informed medicine. When applying evidence to inform treatment, I find it reasonable to use a scale of rigor for the evidence—the more potentially dangerous the intervention, the higher the need for rigorous clinical trials before a recommendation is made. A new surgical technique, or a new toxic chemotherapy, for example, would need a high-grade level of evidence—namely several randomized double-blinded studies that have been peer reviewed and replicated elsewhere. To recommend a deep breath for relaxation, this rigor—while still very nice to have—is not essential. We breathe from the moment of birth until the moment we die, so it is indisputable that breathing is safe. Reasonable evidence detailing how precise breath techniques promote certain health benefits may be enough for recommending a trial in a patient. Additionally, such rigor of research for deep breathing is not feasible. A clinical trial can cost hundreds of thousands of dollars. If there is no product to be sold, and no industry to profit from a breathing intervention, researchers may find that all of their proposals and requests for research funds are declined. Some researchers in integrative fields have resorted to raising their own funding by creating crowd-funding platforms and have carried out their work on a shoestring budget by donating hundreds of hours of their time in uncompensated labor. Despite such gargantuan challenges, there is a surprising abundance of high-quality clinical trials in integrative approaches available to inform treatment. This speaks to the dedication of the many researchers and physicians who devote their time to pursuing good, if rather thanklessly.

This protocol has been compiled and informed by available research on the effects of individual natural therapies on CFS and Long COVID. It has been tested and optimized by feedback from several hundreds of patients I have seen over the years with CFS and now Long Haul. I hope that it proves useful to you too. I temper my optimism knowing that no single approach has been rigorously studied in the treatment of Long COVID—in either the conventional or integrative fields. We need more and better research to inform future therapies. But this doesn't mean nothing can be done in the interim.

In the 1980s, the HIV crisis brought about rapid advances in the field of immunology and the treatment of opportunistic infections. Will COVID be the prompt that advances the treatment of CFS and our understanding of its complex physiology? Perhaps, the Long COVID crisis proves to be the human experience that brings some of the holistic approaches long used in integrative medicine from the fringe into mainstream practice. There are strong economic incentives pushing against this evolution. It may well require a tsunami wave of fatigued sufferers around the globe to change the current tides of practice. To what lengths will Long COVID break down walls and stir advances in the treatment of the devastating condition that is chronic fatigue syndrome? The journey has just begun.

INTRODUCTION

The Rise of Pandemics

"Winter is Coming."
George R. R. Martin, *Game of Thrones*

lobal pandemics have been increasing in frequency since their advent in the 14th century. In 2020-2022 we universally experienced the COVID pandemic with an estimated death toll exceeding 18 million by December 2021.[1] One century ago, 50-100 million people died during the Spanish Flu pandemic of 1918-1920. Two hundred years before the Spanish Flu, the bubonic plague, or the "black death," infected communities on the American continent in 1616-1619, brought by settlers who arrived from Europe to colonize the new world. The plague decimated 90% of the indigenous colonies of the American continent, making it much easier for Spanish colonizers to conquer the warrior cultures in Mexico and the Latin American countries. Three hundred years before the discovery of the Americas, the bubonic plague infected the Eurasian continent in 1347-1351 and killed approximately 25 to 50 million people. The physician Galen recorded the first pandemic in 1347. He named the pandemic the bubonic plague because of ulcerations, or "buboes" that appeared on the skin near lymph nodes.

Pandemics historically have originated from animal vectors that could crossover and infect humans. Expansion of civilization and encroachment into natural habitats by deforestation increased the rate of crossover exposure. The bubonic plague transferred the bacterium Yersinia Pestis from rats via tick bites into humans. An influenza strain known as H1N1, transferred from the avian population to humans and became known as the Spanish Flu. The advent of pandemics coincided with increased world travel and the opening of trade routes, making it easier for a new infection to spread to other countries and continents. The opening of the Silk Road and heavy trade between the Europe and Asia facilitated the first pandemic. With increased affordability and fluidity of travel, pandemics have sped up in frequency over the centuries. Therefore, as globalization, industrialization and international travel continue to rise, COVID will not the be last pandemic that we face, but we can likely expect to experience another pandemic in our lifetime. Current analysis already shows that deer are carrying strains of COVID virus and will act as an animal reservoir to fuel future resurgences. The annual winter flu has an animal reservoir in birds. Scientists test migrating birds yearly to analyze the prevalent influenza strains and to inform our annual vaccines with variable success.

Smaller pandemics have occurred as well. In 1968, a pandemic killing an estimated 1 million people worldwide was caused by an influenza A (H3N2) virus of avian origin. In 1957 the H2N2 virus caused another influenza pandemic. The H3N2 virus continues to circulate worldwide as the seasonal influenza A virus. The influenza viruses are unique in that they have not required a vector of transmission, like a tick or a mosquito, but are spread by direct contact with animals.

Pandemics have likely occurred since the beginning of human civilization. Before the 1300s, when international trade routes were built, highly transmissible infections would have been contained in a single isolated population and would have burned out locally. Those infections likely decimated the local communities, but survivors developed natural immunity and the infection spread was self-limited. The mysterious disappearance of large colonies of Vikings is now attributed to ancient poxvirus strains over 1400 years ago that were found in skeletal remains. It is likely that Vikings introduced smallpox to the European continent during the Viking Age as they colonized western and southern Europe. What makes pandemics more dangerous and could explain their rise in frequency is the globalization of trade. The flattening of international boundaries and advances in world travel have eliminated the protective factor of an epidemic possibly burning out locally. International travel has created the ability for viruses to make several rounds around the globe. As they mutate in one population, they become ready to resurface in a distant part of the world on the first international flight.

My grandfather used to tell me stories about barely surviving the Spanish flu pandemic when he was 10. He lost many family members, including his mother. He described how horse carriages passed through the streets and bodies were piled up like firewood, destined for mass graves. I never thought I would experience anything similar. It was my incorrect belief that our advances in technology and medicine would protect us from such horror. Yet today I realize it is precisely our technologic advances that make us vulnerable to the eruption and global spread of infections, both new and old. It is humbling that a small piece of viral protein can bring the world to its knees after 100 years of scientific and medical advancements. With knowledge and preparation, we can be ready to meet the next pandemic challenge.

I work at the University of California, San Francisco Osher Center for Integrative Health as a consultant. Among its functions, our clinic serves as a referral center for CFS, myalgic encephalitis, and now COVID Long Haul. There are similarities between chronic fatigue syndrome and Long Haul that make specialists familiar with treating chronic fatigue well equipped to treat this new syndrome. By the time I see a referral for Long-Haul syndrome, patients have been struggling with symptoms for over a year. While my protocol is effective, the longer someone has had post-viral fatigue, the longer it takes to convince the body's tissues to change their course. It is almost as if the cellular tissues develop "bad habits" that are difficult to correct, and they accept inflammation as the new normal. My aim in this book is to make knowledge of my protocol available to everyone, so it can empower them to implement corrective strategies early on after the first positive COVID test, and hopefully recover faster. In an era where we seek to improve health equity and access, I hope to make this knowledge available to all, so people can get back to living the life they once had.

For those who are fortunate to survive COVID, approximately 1 in 3 will develop symptoms consistent with Long COVID.[2] At the time of this writing, in September 2022, it is estimated the burden of Long COVID affects up to 23 million people in the United States alone, not to mention the larger impact world-wide. Long COVID has been described in the medical literature as COVID PACS or Post-acute COVID-19 syndrome, and as PAC, or Post-acute COVID. People have called it Long COVID, or Long Haul, and the name has stuck. I will refer to the syndrome as Long COVID or Long Haul from now on since this is how it is commonly described. I wrote this book to share my experiences gained while treating chronic fatigue syndrome, then Long COVID, and the lessons I have learned as my understanding of the biology of the virus has grown.

Long-COVID symptoms can vary over time, but often include fatigue, disruption of digestion and bowel function, ongoing shortness of breath, insomnia, anxiety, brain fog, headaches, palpitations, chest pain, changes in blood pressure, dizziness upon standing, and exercise intolerance, to name a few. Other symptoms include clotting complications like strokes or leg clots (known as DVTs), myocarditis and pericarditis, and autoimmune flares, as well as new (de novo) autoimmune syndromes, and neurologic symptoms. According to the CDC, we diagnose Long COVID when symptoms persist beyond four weeks after clearing the infection. Having prior existing inflammatory illnesses, such as diabetes, obesity, or autoimmune illnesses, is a risk factor. But even previously healthy people with no prior health problems can develop Long COVID. Long-COVID symptoms are variable and unique in their manifestation in each person, though fatigue, exertional malaise and brain fog are the most common (Figure 1). Because of the variable presentations, Long COVID is best evaluated by a holistic and personalized approach and may require collaboration between a team of clinical specialists.

Figure 1. COMMON LONG COVID SYMPTOMS

REMAINING SYMPTOMS AFTER MONTH 7 (PREVALENCE >30%)

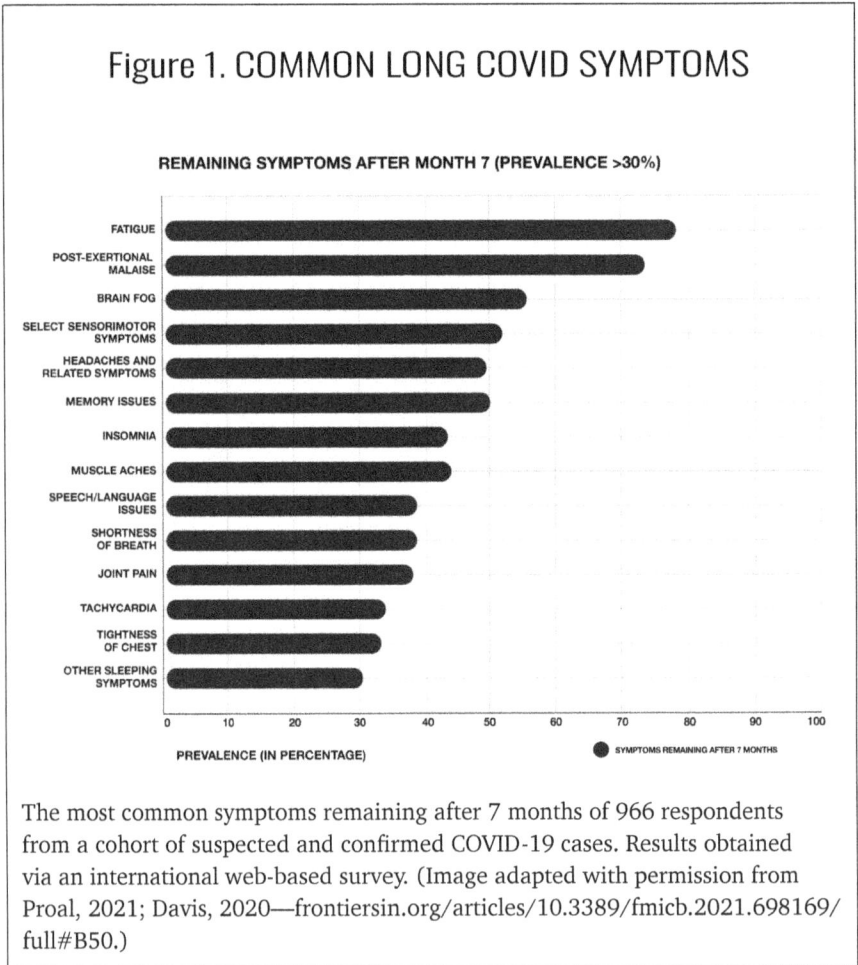

PREVALENCE (IN PERCENTAGE)   ● SYMPTOMS REMAINING AFTER 7 MONTHS

The most common symptoms remaining after 7 months of 966 respondents from a cohort of suspected and confirmed COVID-19 cases. Results obtained via an international web-based survey. (Image adapted with permission from Proal, 2021; Davis, 2020—frontiersin.org/articles/10.3389/fmicb.2021.698169/full#B50.)

Many of the symptoms of Long Haul, or any post-viral fatigue for that matter, are largely because of a failed resolution of the inflammatory surge that was necessary for the immune system to combat the virus. In a body that is not inflamed, a viral infection will generate an inflammatory reaction called an "inflammasome." This inflammasome will turn on the immune system to fight off the virus. Once the virus clears, pathways that resolve inflammation called "resolvins" activate and things return to normal. The fatigue, body aches, temperature changes and headaches disappear, and the person can resume their normal activities. If a pre-existing condition is present which creates ongoing inflammation, the immune system may have a hard time fully resolving inflammation after the virus is gone, and the symptoms of fatigue, headaches, and feelings of un-wellness persist. Inflammation is thus the driving factor for most post-viral syndromes. In upcoming chapters, I will describe how to adopt an anti-inflammatory lifestyle and supplements which support the resolution of inflammation.

The second factor to consider is toxin increase. Infection causes increased cellular death, and both the infection and inflammatory surge will create a toxic burden for the body. The successful killing of viruses and virus-infected cells cause increased toxin debris, cellular debris, and reactive oxygen species (ROS). This results in an increased burden for the detoxifying organs of the body, namely the liver and kidneys. The liver detoxifies reactive oxygen species and free radicals by a couple of mechanisms, the main one being the glutathione pathway. Glutathione is a tripeptide made by the liver which binds free radicals and toxins, neutralizing them in the process. When glutathione binds a toxin, the toxin becomes inert and it is more easily eliminated via either urine or feces. When glutathione binds free radicals, it converts them into water. Therefore, besides resolving inflammation, it is important to support the liver. The kidneys can be supported by drinking more water. Toxins produced while killing microbes cause the Herxheimer reaction or what I like to call "die off." Herxheimer reactions are short-term detoxification reactions in the body, and they produce flu-like symptoms including headache, nausea, joint and muscle pain, body aches, and malaise. Die-off feels like much like a hangover with some flu-like symptoms. One way to reduce Herxheimer reactions in the body is to support detoxification while you are being treated for an infection.

The liver produces another important enzyme called aldehyde dehydrogenase, or ALDH. This enzyme is involved in detoxifying histamine and alcohol, and it is important in regulation of histamine-mediated inflammation. We will address detoxification in the chapter on toxins.

Post-viral fatigue is nothing new. Annual viruses such as Influenza, or the Epstein-Barr virus have caused post-infectious symptoms long after the infection has resolved. Therefore, many of the tools that I will present to you for COVID recovery can apply to many viral illnesses. COVID recovery is a little different, though. The post-viral syndrome following COVID infection seems to be more severe, lingers for a longer period, and seems to affect more organs. COVID has the special ability to kick the hornet's nest of any prior existing conditions to make them flare. I have found that if patients had a pre-existing condition in a particular organ, that this condition flared and formed part of their unique constellation of COVID Long-Haul syndrome. For example, patients with underlying lung inflammation like mild asthma may have inflammation settle in the lungs and have prolonged cough or shortness of breath. Patients who may have had a heart attack in the pre-existing year before developing COVID may develop myocarditis. Patients who have arthritis may develop more joint pain. People who have pre-existing autoimmune conditions may experience a flare in their condition because the immune system remains strongly activated long after the COVID infection has resolved. The challenge COVID presents to the immune system can lead a window of opportunity for other existing viruses, like EBV or herpes viruses, to reactivate. COVID may even cause changes in the immune environment, leading to the development of "de-novo" or new autoimmunity.[3]

Finally, COVID inflammation can dysregulate the central nervous system via inflammation in brain regulatory centers. We have twelve cranial nerves in our brain, and one, cranial nerve X, is deeply affected. Cranial nerve X is better known as the vagus nerve. Vago in Latin means "wanderer," and this word aptly describes it since the vagus is the only nerve that travels throughout the front and center of our body. After the vagus nerve leaves the safety net of the brain, it connects to various organs along the way: the voice-box, the lungs, heart, diaphragm, stomach, bowels, liver, spleen, and kidneys. Vagal outflow tracts present in all these organs help to maintain optimal function of the organs and to reduce inflammation in those organs. The vagus is exquisitely sensitive to inflammatory surges such as those caused by COVID, and it can become dysregulated. When the vagal tone weakens, any of these organs can malfunction. The dysregulation promotes more inflammation, and now you have a looped inflammation cycle that is hard to break. Therefore, vagal toning, or "strengthening," is key in the recovery process.

Besides organ regulation, the vagus regulates our autonomic system (ANS). The ANS has two states: "fight or flight" on one end and the "rested, fed, and relaxed" state on the other end. It is not uncommon for people with Long COVID to have increased anxiety, a sense of dread, insomnia, tachycardia, palpitations; all symptoms of a fight-or-flight response that is permanently activated. The vagus acts much like a brake pad on the fight-or-flight response. Have you ever driven a car with old brake pads and tried to stop at a stop sign? The car keeps moving and is hard to control. When the vagal tone weakens, fight-or-flight runs rampant, much the same way the old car won't stop. Vagal dystonia results in a constant state of heightened alertness and stress. Coming back to the car analogy, a car that is driven too hard wastes precious gasoline. Similarly, heightened stress physiology contributes to fatigue by wasting precious, energetic resources. I will address vagal toning techniques in the neuroinflammation chapter.

Generally, I find that causes of fatigue fall into one of four big categorical buckets: too much inflammation, too many toxins, nutrient deficiencies, and/or too much stress physiology. It is helpful to think of these four buckets as you read this book and as we create a plan to address them in subsequent chapters. (See Figure 2. The Four Drivers of Fatigue.)

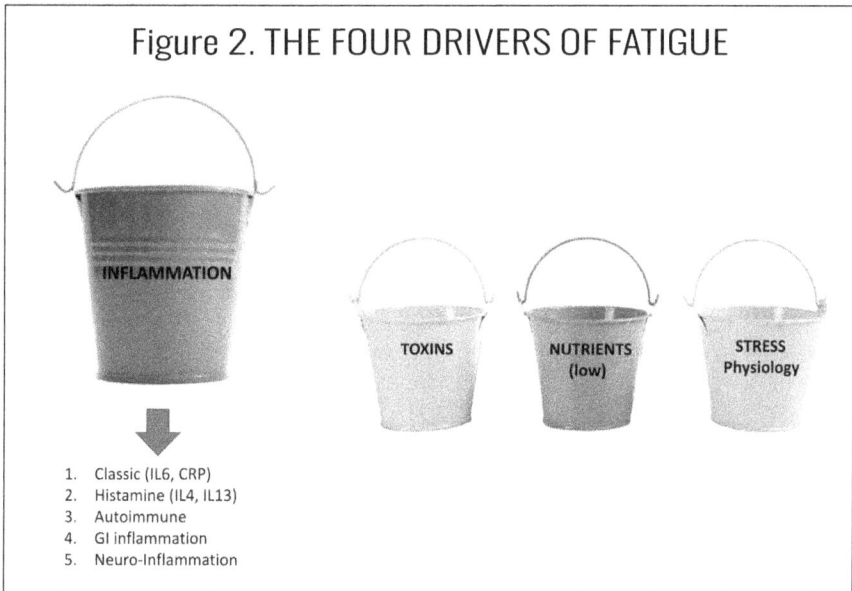

Figure 2. THE FOUR DRIVERS OF FATIGUE

INFLAMMATION

TOXINS

NUTRIENTS (low)

STRESS Physiology

1. Classic (IL6, CRP)
2. Histamine (IL4, IL13)
3. Autoimmune
4. GI inflammation
5. Neuro-Inflammation

I hope that by reading this book you will become equipped with the tools to improve your health and support a full recovery from COVID should you be exposed to it. Preventing Long Haul may become a part of your permanent pandemic toolbox after reading this guide. By making this knowledge widely available, I hope to give everyone a fighting chance against Long COVID and decrease the lingering burden of disabling fatigue experienced by COVID survivors.

Summary

- Pandemics have been rising in frequency ever since the first recorded pandemic in the 14th century, the bubonic plague, also known as the "black death."
- Globalization, deforestation, and increases in world travel contribute to the increase in frequency of pandemics, making it likely we will see another pandemic in our lifetime.

- Long COVID is present when post-viral symptoms are present four weeks beyond COVID recovery. Symptoms of Long COVID commonly include fatigue, exercise intolerance, and brain fog, but can include many other symptoms and affect many organs.
- Fatigue generally falls under four big buckets: inflammation, toxins, nutrient deficiencies, and stress physiology.
- Inflammation is the biggest driver of Long-COVID symptoms and is large enough to contain five subcategories. Therefore, addressing inflammation is key in decreasing symptoms of post-viral fatigue.

CHAPTER 1

Prevention

"An ounce of prevention is worth a pound of cure."
Benjamin Franklin

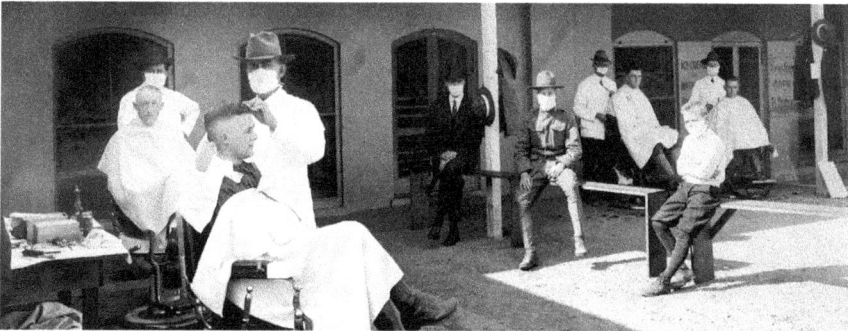

An open-air barbershop. Public events were encouraged to be held outdoors to hinder the spread of the disease during the influenza epidemic. Photographed at the University of California, Berkeley, in 1919. National archives ID 26428662. Public domain.

Some advantages of our current pandemic compared to the prior ones have been the scientific advances in medicine, including DNA sequencing technology, the availability of vaccines, and the rapid development of new anti-viral medications. Although our science cannot prevent the onset of a pandemic, tools have emerged for prevention and protection that were not available before. I was very interested in discovering the above image from the Spanish Flu pandemic, and to know that we are not that much different today apart from the rapid development of vaccines and anti-viral medications.

The best way to prevent COVID Long Haul is to prevent getting COVID in the first place. In vaccinated individuals, even in those who get COVID after vaccination, there is a much lower risk for subsequent Long-Haul syndrome. Vaccination also has been highly effective at preventing death and hospitalization.[4]

Reading this book should not dissuade people from getting protective vaccination, or falsely reassure them that if they get COVID and take supplements, they will be okay. COVID is associated with significant disease burden, mortality, and functional impairment. The immune response and adverse consequences to the COVID virus in the unvaccinated differs from the immune response in someone who gets the vaccine and subsequently becomes infected with COVID. I write this book to help those infected, or in recovery, to be supported in their healing regardless of vaccine status. In the final chapter, I will discuss how to prepare your body for the vaccine and how to reduce post-vaccine side effects.

The COVID vaccine causes the immune system to generate a precise antibody to a single protein, the spike-(S)-protein, which is the gateway of entry for the virus. We measure spike protein antibodies when we test response to the vaccine. Natural infection, on the other hand, elicits the generation of multiple antibodies, including nucleocapsid (N) protein, envelope protein,

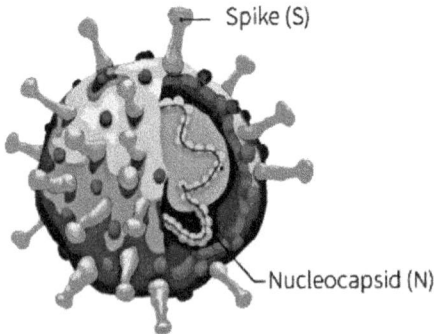

Figure 3. SARS-COV2-VIRUS

Spike (S)

Nucleocapsid (N)

Spike (S): Antibodies to the spike protein are produced after vaccination[1-3]

Nucleocapsid (N): Antibodies to Nucleocapsid identify individuals who have had a recent or prior COVID-19 infection, but are not useful for detecting antibodies elicited by currently available SARS-CoV-2 vaccines.

Adapted with permission from www.pennmedicine.org/updates/blogs/penn-physician-blog/2020/august/covid19-vaccine-research-at-penn-searching-for-covid-immunity/

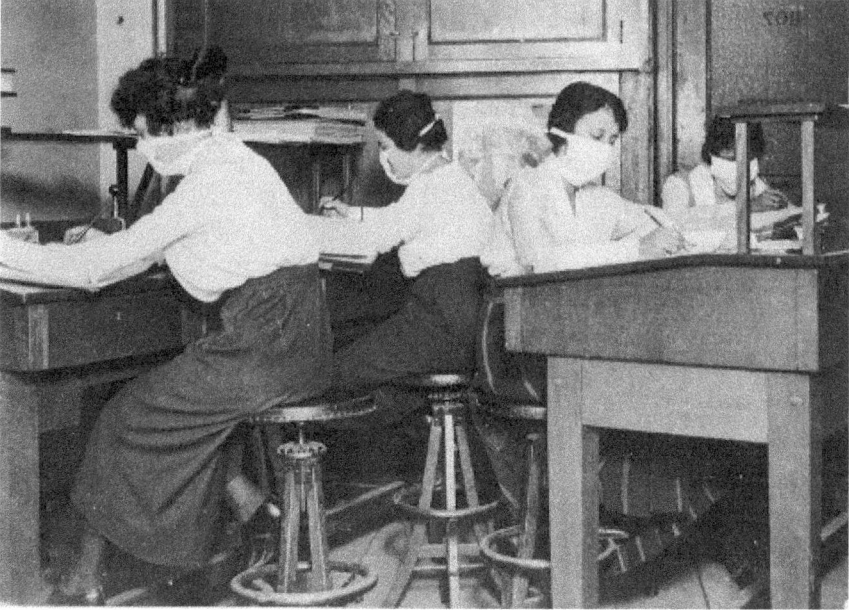

Female clerks in New York City wear masks at work. National archives id 45499337. Public domain.

(I) and membrane (M) protein antibodies. This messier process can increase the chance that these antibodies will cross react with self-tissues and generate an auto-immune process.[5]

You might think: "I'm better off getting the real thing." However, that conclusion would be incorrect. Studies of COVID antibody duration in vaccinated individuals as opposed to immunity gained from natural infection shows that vaccinated individuals have longer lasting circulating protective antibodies. Natural immunity carries a higher risk of developing Long-Haul symptoms. Not to mention a much higher risk of hospitalization and even death. Whether you had the good fortune to have a shot or two on your arm before you got COVID, or if you developed the infection without the vaccine's protection, this book should help speed up your recovery. Ideally, starting this protocol while still infected or early in the recovery is best. The timeline to recovery should be quick in this scenario. The longer the Long-COVID syndrome has been present, the slower you can expect the recovery process to be. Regardless of where you are in your recovery, following these guidelines will accelerate your healing and improve your state of function.

Masks have been shown to be effective barriers to COVID exposure. I get it, mask fatigue is real! However, there are several studies that show wearing masks in indoor or high exposure areas reduces the risk of transmission.

Remember, the best way to avoid Long-COVID is to avoid getting infected in the first place! Vaccination decreases the risk of Long-COVID after infection and it is a convincing reason to consider vaccination and booster shots.

Summary

- Vaccines are highly effective against death, severe COVID illness, and hospitalization.
- Vaccines are protective against Long COVID and are another reason to consider vaccination, though they are not 100% protective for Long COVID.
- The best way to avoid getting Long COVID is to not get COVID in the first place.
- Consider wearing masks in high-risk situations even if vaccinated and boosted, even though mask fatigue is real!

CHAPTER 2

Inflammation is One of the Key Drivers of Long-Haul Symptoms

Dreading that climax of all human ills
the inflammation of his weekly bills.
Lord Byron

The Fatigue-Inflammation Axis

Though symptoms of Long COVID vary in each person, fatigue is the most common symptom reported. Generally, I find that fatigue falls under four categorical buckets, with inflammation being the biggest driver of fatigue. Therefore, bucket number one is inflammation, and it is such a large bucket that it contains five separate divisions: 1) classic inflammation, 2) histamine-mediated inflammation, 3) auto-immune inflammation, 4) gastrointestinal inflammation and 5) neuroinflammation. Immune dysfunction often coexists with frequent or chronic infections, which drives more inflammation. Immune dysfunction can result from autoimmunity, or an immune system that has been activated for so long that it saves energy by downregulating its function. Besides the gigantic bucket that is inflammation, there are three more buckets that contribute to fatigue: too many toxins (bucket two), nutrient deficiencies (bucket three), and high stress physiology (bucket four). We will address them in subsequent chapters.

Figure 4. THE FATIGUE-INFLAMMATION AXIS

1. Classic (IL-6, ↑CRP)
2. Histamine (IL-4, IL-13)
3. Autoimmune (IL-6, IL-17)
4. Neuro-Inflammation
   (Migraines, brain fog)
5. GI inflammation (IBD, IBS,
   food sensitivity)

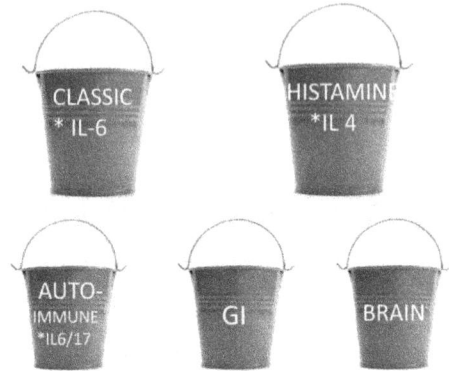

CLASSIC * IL-6

HISTAMINE *IL 4

AUTO-IMMUNE *IL6/17

GI

BRAIN

Classic inflammation is what we normally believe inflammation to be—the achy muscles or joint pains you feel when you are fighting a virus are symptoms from classic inflammation. Classic inflammation is driven by interleukin 6, a chemical signal that activates the immune system and is indirectly measured by the serum C-reactive protein assay (CRP). We see during an infection that CRP goes up, then normalizes after the virus is gone. The second type of inflammation, histamine-mediated inflammation, is usually due to increased interleukin 4, and interleukin 13. These cytokines drive increased histamine release in the body, and they are indirectly measured by checking histamine or tryptase levels in the blood. Autoimmunity is driven by interleukin 6 and interleukin 17. Autoimmunity can often be measured by checking levels of autoantibodies, and these will vary depending on the organ that is being affected. Gastrointestinal inflammation sometimes can be detected by an elevated fecal calprotectin or seen in procedures such as an endoscopy or colonoscopy, but there are more subtle forms of inflammation that can be harder to capture unless you use specialized testing such as microbiome testing. They include secretory IgA and intestinal zonulin markers. Neuroinflammation can be even more challenging to measure, and it usually manifests as either pain or dysfunction of the brain, such as headaches or brain fog. Neuroinflammation can be present even when a brain scan such as an MRI or CT scan is completely normal. You can see why Long-Haul symptoms vary so much between one person and another, since there are many pathways that can generate inflammation. You can also see how this complexity would pose a taxing diagnostic challenge to any clinician.

Patients who have chronic fatigue can have inflammation stemming from one bucket, and one inflammatory category. Other patients have several buckets active, and more than one type of inflammatory drive active all at once. It may take an expert clinician well versed in chronic fatigue to unravel all the contributing causes, and to address each bucket systematically. These patients may benefit from a team of physicians collaborating in their care.

Inflammation is probably one of the largest drivers of all chronic illnesses. However, inflammation isn't always bad for you. Short-term inflammation serves to activate your immune system so it can fight off an infection. Self-limited inflammation, such as that caused by exercise, can help build muscle and activate mechanisms of cellular repair and regeneration. This type of inflammation is called "hormesis" and it is a type of adaptive or "good" stress. Hormetic stress stimulates re-building of muscle and collagen, cellular regeneration, and a healing response after exercise.

The inflammation that needs to be addressed here is long-term, unresolved chronic inflammation. Long-term inflammation can affect everything negatively from head to toe, and it speeds up the aging of the organs. Too much inflammation in the brain accelerates memory loss and causes cognitive dysfunction. Inflammation in the circulatory system can cause hardening of the arteries and activates platelet adhesion. Platelet adhesion is when activated platelets develop Velcro-like qualities, and this activation can cause coronary plaque formation, heart disease, stroke, or blood clots. Inflammation of the joints over time will lead to arthritis and degenerative joint disease. High systemic inflammation can contribute to lowered immunity, increased susceptibility to frequent viral infections, viral reactivations, and fatigue, therefore aging the immune system. Inflammation, therefore, contributes to rapid aging of the entire body. This process has been termed "inflammaging." If you learn nothing in this book except how to lower inflammation in your body, you will have achieved a positive impact on your long-term health.

In a healthy, uninflamed body, exposure to an infection with a virus or bacteria will activate the inflammasome pathway. Immune cells called T-helper type 1 (Th1) cells release inflammatory chemicals, also known as cytokines, including type 1 interferon, and this activates the immune system's "fight" response. Once the infection has successfully cleared from the body, a new mechanism activates that resolves that inflammation back to the baseline state. Anti-inflammatory cytokines mediate this change, known as "resolvins." Interferon levels go down and disappear. In such a curve, a person feels well at baseline, then feels fatigued and achy during an infection. Once the infection clears, they return to their original state of health.

But what happens in a scenario where there is a failure to resolve inflammation back to the pre-infection state? Here, inflammation lowers after the infection clears, but it does not completely resolve. Health does not return to baseline even after the signs of the infection are over. This can lead to symptoms of post-viral fatigue or Long-COVID.

In this scenario, a person has a long-standing health condition which causes the body to have high chronic inflammation before the infection. The pre-existing inflammation generates a sluggish interferon response. The virus can replicate for longer before being suppressed by the immune system, causing more organ damage along the way. It is more difficult to resolve the inflammation afterwards. Conditions that have been associated with increased systemic inflammation run the gamut. Diabetes, obesity, heart disease, gout, arthritis, autoimmune conditions, inflammatory bowel disease, sarcoidosis, hypoxic lung diseases like lung fibrosis and chronic obstructive lung disease, as well as chronic infections like untreated hepatitis, are all associated with chronic inflammation. Figure 5 shows these two separate scenarios.

I give credit to Dr. Yanuck for being one of the first immunology experts

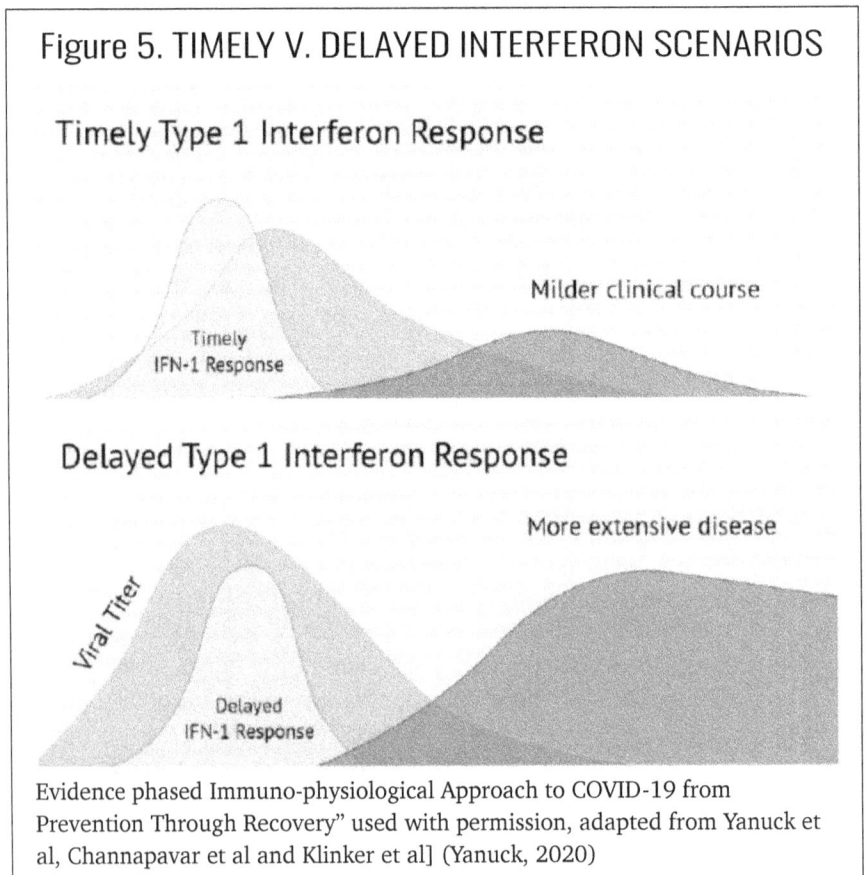

Figure 5. TIMELY V. DELAYED INTERFERON SCENARIOS

Timely Type 1 Interferon Response

Milder clinical course

Timely
IFN-1 Response

Delayed Type 1 Interferon Response

More extensive disease

Viral Titer

Delayed
IFN-1 Response

Evidence phased Immuno-physiological Approach to COVID-19 from Prevention Through Recovery" used with permission, adapted from Yanuck et al, Channapavar et al and Klinker et al] (Yanuck, 2020)

to present a protocol for Long Haul early in the pandemic. I relied on it to inform my early treatment of patients. The article is free to download, and it details a rationale for supporting the body from prevention through recovery. Although the article is written for medical professionals, figures 1-3 are highly informative, and I have included them in this chapter with permission.[6]

COVID is so good at increasing inflammation, in fact, it has been associated with "cytokine storm," which is like a tsunami of overwhelming inflammation. In patients hospitalized with severe COVID and acute respiratory distress syndrome (ARDS), the inflammatory cytokines brought patients near a fatality risk threshold. Thus, inflammation, not the virus, causes organ failure (See Figure 6). The lungs, kidneys, brain, and heart all collapse like dominoes and patients require life support when that happens. A 2020 study found that early administration of high potency anti-inflammatory steroids reduced this cytokine storm and improved survival, decreasing the need for life support and intensive care. This major

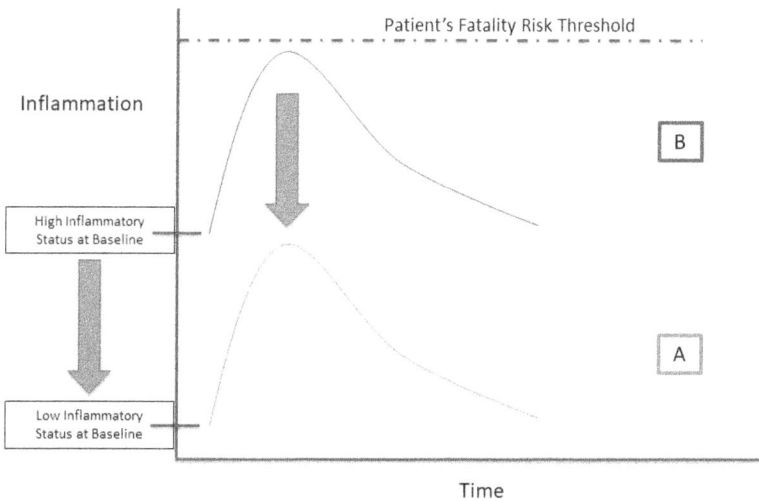

Figure 6. INFLAMMATION/FATALITY CURVE

In A, patient's baseline inflammation is low. Cytokine response to the virus increases inflammation, and this is accommodated by the patient's biology. In B, patient's baseline inflammation is higher. The same incremental inflammatory cytokine response to the virus increases risk of developing ARDS, increasing fatality risk. Ref: Yanuck: "Evidence phased Immuno-physiological Approach to COVID-19 from Prevention Through Recovery." Used with permission.

discovery led to better care for COVID patients and improved survival rates early in the pandemic.[7]

Therefore, the first bucket of Long COVID that needs to be addressed is unresolved inflammation. Fortunately, there are several ways to lower inflammation besides taking steroids. In my first visit with a patient with Long Haul, I take time and effort to educate them on the anti-inflammatory diet. I spend almost an hour teaching and answering questions because proper nutrition is essential to recovery. This is often surprising to patients because doctors rarely talk about diet. Some patients even mistake me for dietician. I prioritize nutrition because the anti-inflammatory diet is the foundation without which the anti-inflammatory supplements simply won't work. Supplements alone cannot overcome an inflammatory diet and lifestyle.

In my career as an integrative medicine physician, I have been amazed at the power of proper nutrition, when combined with carefully selected supplements. In the next chapter we will go over the foundations of the anti-inflammatory diet.

Summary

- Unresolved inflammation is one of the key drivers of Long-COVID symptoms and it is the first bucket that needs to be addressed in chronic fatigue.
- Inflammation is a big enough bucket that it contains five subcategories:
  1 Classic inflammation
  2 Histamine-mediated inflammation
  3 Autoimmune inflammation
  4 Gastrointestinal inflammation.
  5 Neuroinflammation
- The anti-inflammatory diet, combined with carefully chosen targeted supplements, can have profound effects on lowering inflammation in the body and it will be discussed in the next chapter.

CHAPTER 3

The Anti-Inflammatory Diet

"Let food be thy medicine, and medicine thy food."
Hippocrates, Greek physician, and the founder of medicine, 460 BC–375 BC

"*Quod ali cibus est aliis fuat acre venenum.*"
(What is food for one man may be bitter poison to others)
Roman poet and philosopher Titus Lucretius Carus, 99 BC–55 BC

Much has been written and much has been said about what diet is best and which diet should be consumed. Many books have been written by medical doctors who contradict each other's recommendations. Diet fads have come and gone leaving people confused and exhausted about figuring out what foods they should eat. Not surprisingly, many have simply given up. Some may swear by a diet that turned their life around completely, gave them energy, and helped them lose unwanted weight. Others may have tried the same diet but felt worse off. So perhaps I should start this chapter by pre-emptively making a statement of caution: Diet is not a one-size-fits-all approach. This is main reason diet fads surge and fade. Be very careful of anyone, even if this person is a physician, who adopts a militant approach or makes sweeping dietary recommendations for everyone. By the sheer enormity of biological, genetic, and epigenetic diversity, such a totalitarian statement is by logic simplistic, reductionistic, and cannot be objectively true for every person. One person's treasured food may well be another person's poison.

Hippocrates, widely considered the father of medicine, keenly observed a connection between food and health and created the well-known aphorism "Let food be thy medicine." Another "influencer" of the times was the roman poet Titus Lucretius, widely known to be Hellenistic (meaning *Greek*) and Epicurean. An epicure is someone who loved food of all types and today would be considered a "foodie." Lucretius countered that not everyone could benefit from the same diet.

Hippocrates advocated for smaller portions, intermittent fasting, and a plant-based diet filled with "anything that comes from Mother Earth without man's intervention like fruits, vegetables, nuts and seeds." The poet Lucretius was Hellenistic, and one can imagine, probably enjoyed a good deal of wine and red meat, as the Romans and Greeks did in those days. He theorized living organisms survived because of the commensurate relationship between their strength, speed, or intellect and the external dynamics of their environment.

It is telling to note that Lucretius is thought to have died at 44, while Hippocrates is thought to have lived beyond the age of 104. Though they did not live in the same century, it would have been fun to have watched Hippocrates and Lucretius meet and debate passionately the pros and cons of opposite dietary choices. However, while Hippocrates made an astute connection between different dietary choices and subsequently benefitted from selecting the better food choices, poor Lucretius was not entirely wrong.

There are dietary guidelines we can indeed generalize. Junk foods like refined sugar, fried foods, highly processed foods, and processed meats have well documented negative impacts on the body, and most folks are educated enough about diet to know that already. Even those who still choose to eat those foods, because of convenience, budget, or lack of time, know they probably should eat more greens to improve their nutrition. But diet is not a one-size fits-all concept. When I evaluate patients in the clinic, I am applying my understanding of their individual biology to guide my personalized dietary recommendations. Indeed, I normally recommend diet and supplements on our second visit, after carrying out additional testing to guide my choices. We are genetically unique and have individual nutritional needs. We have genetic and epigenetic contributions which influence how we interact with our environment and with our food. Case in point: My Italian grandfather lived a healthy life and died at the grand old age of 105, with his intelligence and memory fully intact. He was a bit like Hippocrates, and astute enough to restrict his intake of meat as he advanced into old age by eating a mostly a vegetarian diet. In fact, he was one week shy of celebrating 105 when he died in his sleep, so he was pretty darn close! My Italian grandmother, his wife, was the kindest woman and an exquisite cook, but she was chronically ill and died at 77. Her life was plagued with health issues, several cancers, heart attacks and dementia before she died. She walked slowly, looked swollen, and I remember how she always looked fatigued. I subsequently learned that there is a genetic variant in my mother's family that increases the risk of celiac disease, which I suspect she had. Several members in my family have now been diagnosed with celiac disease, including myself. The same Italian diet that gave my grandfather a healthy long life probably caused my grandmother to have a shortened life plagued with health challenges. "One man's meat is another man's poison" therefore rings true, although poor Lucretius seemed to shorten his life with his lifestyle choices and excesses.

For this reason, I do not prescribe the same diet to all my patients. Sometimes I will conduct a nutrigenomics evaluation to further refine diet and supplement recommendations. Despite this, there is abundant data to support a plant-based diet rich in anti-inflammatory foods such as the omega-3 fats, rich in antioxidants, and which avoids pro-inflammatory foods. This is the foundation upon which I build a more individualized approach for each patient. This diet is called the Anti-Inflammatory diet, and it is largely based on studies on the Mediterranean Diet and blue zones in the world. Blue zones are locations throughout the world where there is an unusually high number of healthy centenarians, much like my grandpa.

I credit Dr. Dean Ornish for initiating the scientific studies to further our understanding of how diet affects outcomes in inflammatory diseases and for initiating the dialogue in the world of medical science, which until then focused only on drug therapies. In 1998, Dr. Ornish published the first 5-year longitudinal study proving that a plant-based diet can reverse cardiovascular health outcomes in a mostly male population with heart disease.[8] I will place this caveat: Most clinical studies on heart disease are largely skewed toward a white male population. Making broad applications of these studies towards minorities and women may be overly simplistic. There is a lot of bias in medical research which excludes the health concerns of minorities and women. Women have unique nutritional challenges in my experience. In my practice, I have seen many women plagued by nutritional deficits not normally encountered in men, such as chronic iron deficiency. A strict vegetarian diet may make it more challenging for them to fulfill their nutritional needs. Women also have a greater tendency for several vitamin deficiencies in large part because of consumption of fewer calories. The standard caloric consumption for women is 1200-1500 kcal, whereas men often consume double this amount. Therefore, there are fewer opportunities to get sufficient nutrients from a much smaller intake of food, by sheer volume of intake. Commonly used medications such as birth control pills can negatively impact absorption and utilization of B vitamins among other nutrients.[9] We need more nutritional studies incorporating equity and diversity to provide a clearer picture of what recommendations can be applied to minority populations and women's health.

Studies into blue zones confirm that plant-based, Mediterranean diets rich in omega-3 fatty acids, plant polyphenols, antioxidants, and reduced animal proteins led to longer and healthier lives as documented by an increased number of healthy centenarians in that population. The Mediterranean diet is my template for the anti-inflammatory diet because evidence strongly backs it across several countries and populations.

I will now go over this diet in detail for you, the same way I would if I were seeing you in my office for a consultation.

When I see patients for the second visit, I review their labs and explain the anti-inflammatory diet with any notable modifications which can be helpful. I share with them Dr. Andrew Weil's anti-inflammatory food pyramid seen below in Figure 7. It is available for free download in his website.[10]

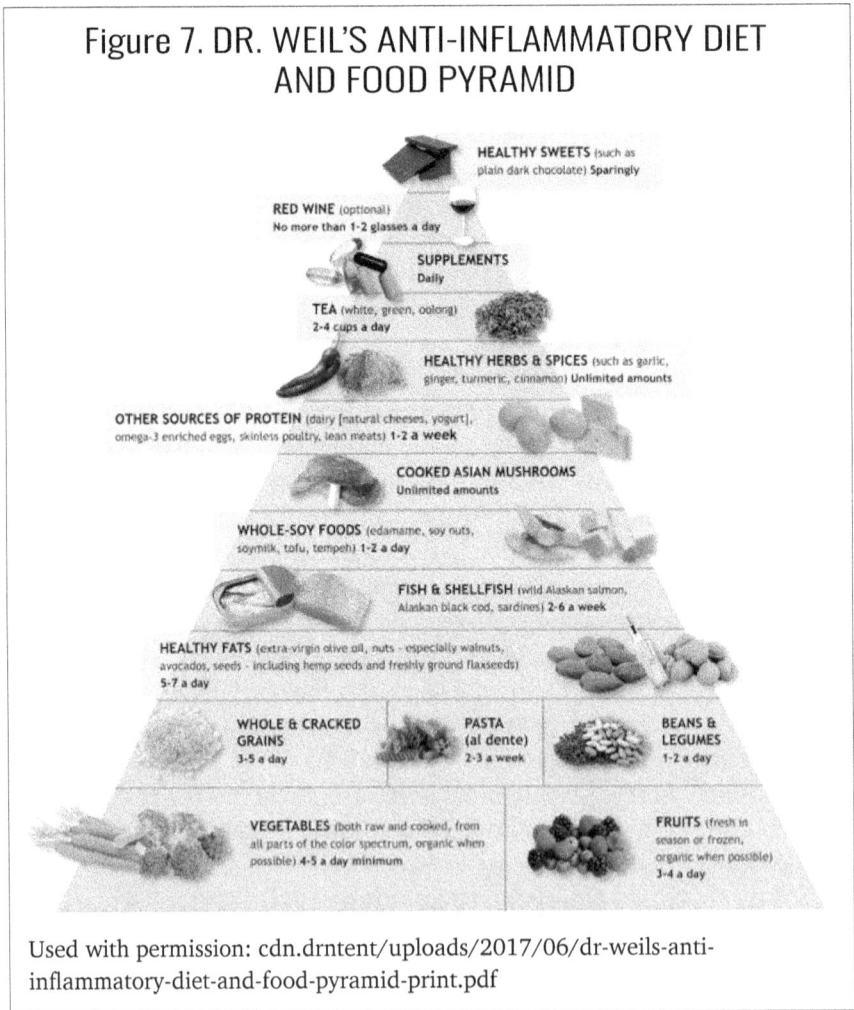

Figure 7. DR. WEIL'S ANTI-INFLAMMATORY DIET AND FOOD PYRAMID

Used with permission: cdn.drntent/uploads/2017/06/dr-weils-anti-inflammatory-diet-and-food-pyramid-print.pdf

I give Dr. Weil credit for continuing the conversation started by Dr. Ornish in the medical field, and for bringing Integrative Medicine to the United States by launching the first specialty fellowship in the University of Arizona. In Integrative Medicine, the Hippocratic Oath of the importance of diet in health and disease is taken seriously and is a foundational part of training. If you have never heard of a doctor speak of diet to manage your disease, it's because they do not teach conventionally trained doctors much about nutrition in medical school. The training I received in nutrition came from my fellowship in Integrative Medicine and from continuous education in this field.

Let's begin from the bottom of the pyramid and work our way up.

Healthy Food Pyramid

Superfood Group #1: Cruciferous Vegetables

The diet emphasizes 5 servings of vegetables daily, and I emphasize the importance of cruciferous vegetables because of their anti-inflammatory properties. The nutrient that gives cruciferous vegetables like broccoli their super-power is sulforaphane. Sulforaphane has a wealth of clinical studies and science that demonstrate both its anti-inflammatory and anti-cancer properties.[11]

Sulforaphanes found in the cruciferous family are what I like to call "nature's steroids." While steroids are the most powerful anti-inflammatories known in western medicine, severe side effects plague them and they are dangerous for long-term use. Steroids kill natural killer cells and thymocytes, known as T cells, both important components of our cell-mediated immunity and our humoral immunity. Steroids are powerful because they enter the cells and change how proteins are made inside the cell by ribosomes. Sulforaphanes can enter the nucleus of a cell and change expression of the inflammatory cytokines, so they are just as powerful, but have none of the side effects associated with steroids. There has been a lot of misinformation about the impact of cruciferous vegetables on the thyroid, and I would like to dispel that myth. Cruciferous vegetables will not damage your thyroid. This family of vegetables contains compounds called goitrogens, which, in high doses, can interfere with iodine uptake in the thyroid. Those doses would have to be much higher than what one gets in the typical western diet. Diets deficient in iodine can become problematic, and this issue is seen in countries with low table salt intake. As of 2020, 124 countries have legislation for mandatory salt iodization, including the United States, and 21 have legislation allowing voluntary iodization. As a result, 88% of the global population uses iodized salt. In the 21 countries in the world where iodized salt is optional, there could be an iodine deficiency. You can look up the 21 countries that have low dietary iodized salt intake in *European Journal of Endocrinology* (doi.org/10.1530/EJE-21-0171).[12] Cooking cruciferous vegetables decreases goitrogen content as well, though cooking also reduces beneficial sulforaphane content, so I do not recommend overcooking this family of vegetables.

If you use table salt, your diet is likely rich in iodine. The high use of table salt in most commercially prepared meals makes iodine deficiency rare in the United States. I recommend cruciferous vegetables for all my patients with hypothyroidism, making sure they are getting enough iodine from dietary sources like table salt, or seaweed intake. It makes no sense to deprive folks of this plant's superpower. Sulforaphanes from vegetables such as broccoli and broccoli sprouts are an essential ingredient in my detoxification and immune modulation work with chronically ill patients.

Superfood Group #2: Berries

Berries get their superpower from a polyphenol called "anthocyanin." Cyanin in Latin means blue, so the darker blue and purple-colored berries have a higher content of this nutrient. Anthocyanins are powerful antioxidants, and whenever you want to lower inflammation in the body, remember to think of lowering oxidative load as well. Antioxidants and anti-inflammatory agents are the right and left hand needed to lower inflammation. Berries are also low in sugar, which is good since high intake of sugar is pro-inflammatory. Another superfood fruit is pomegranate seeds, which contain high amounts polyphenols, including epigallic acid, urolithin A, besides other antioxidants which support hormone detoxification. Urolithin supports cellular regeneration. Pomegranate's high phenolic content has been studied in prostate health and it supports estrogen detoxification. For this reason, its ruby gem seeds are widely known as the "red gems of immortality" in Asian cultures because of their numerous health benefits. I recommend eating five seeds daily, and they can be purchased frozen and de-seeded in most supermarkets for ease.[13] I recommend avoiding all juices, including pomegranate juice, due to their higher sugar content.

Grains

Although not a superfood, I recommend choosing whole grains over refined grains in this food group. Complex carbohydrates found in whole grains give the body sustained energy and do not cause the sugar crashes seen in more refined foods. I recommend whole-grain breads, and brown rice instead of white rice, because of their lower glycemic impact on the body. Refined sugars like white flower and table sugar create a high glucose spike in the blood-stream, known as the glycemic load, and cause excess insulin to be released. This chemistry stimulates the production of IFG-1 (insulin-like growth factor beta), and frequent spikes in IGF-1 have been associated with increased inflammation. It is one reason we consider diabetes to be a pro-inflammatory condition. However, you don't have to be diabetic to have sugar-induced inflammation. Consuming too much sugar or eating highly refined foods can have similar inflammatory effects on the body. Grains can be problematic for a subgroup of people with underlying gastrointestinal inflammatory disease or autoimmune diseases, who may develop an intolerance to gluten or other grains. If you feel you might fit this category, I recommend consultation with a functional nutritionist to determine which foods are safe to incorporate in your diet. For this reason, sugar is one of my foods listed in the "evil triad" of inflammation. If you are wondering which foods are high in sugar, like some of the sweeter fruits, I recommend purchasing the "glycemic load index" book, which lists the glycemic index of all foods. You want to pick foods and fruits with a glycemic index of 40 and below as much as possible.[14]

Figure 8. GLYCEMIC LOAD COUNTER

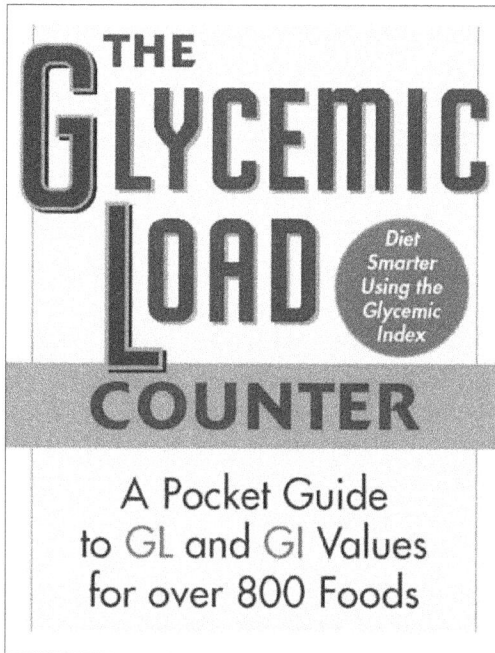

THE GLYCEMIC LOAD COUNTER

Diet Smarter Using the Glycemic Index

A Pocket Guide to GL and GI Values for over 800 Foods

Mabel Blades, *The Glycemic Load Counter: A Pocket Guide*

Beans and Legumes

Beans can be an excellent source of complex carbohydrates, minerals, and black beans are an excellent source of plant-based iron. Legumes and beans can be problematic for the same subset of folks that may be sensitive to grains, so I recommend soaking and pressure-cooking all beans to reduce lectin content. Consider elimination of kidney beans if you have either a gastrointestinal or other autoimmune disease, since kidney beans have the highest inflammatory lectin content.

Superfood Group #3: Omega-3 Oils (ALA)

The western diet—high in animal meats, dairy and vegetable cooking oils—is high in omega-6 fats while low in omega-3 fats. To decrease inflammation, find ways to increase your consumption of omega-3 fats, while reducing the consumption of omega-6 fats. One way to do this is to increase your intake of omega-3 rich foods like nuts and seeds. Walnuts have the highest omega-3 content of all nuts. Flax seeds, hemp, avocados and perilla oil or borage oil are excellent sources too. Olive oil contains mostly omega-9 (Oleic acid) and a smaller amount of omega-3 (about 15%). Omega-9 is another beneficial oil associated with many anti-inflammatory benefits, including cardiovascular benefits. My favorite oil is perilla oil, because of its superior 50-60% omega-3 content. Perilla oil is a staple in Korean cooking and can be used for low heat cooking. Ahiflower oil also has a balanced blend of omega-3 and some gamma linoleic acid (GLA). GLA is the only anti-inflammatory omega-6 fatty acid, and it is frequently low in inflamed persons.

Superfood Group #4: Omega-3 Oils (EPA and DHA)

Our body's most powerful and bioavailable omega-3's come from deep cold-water oily fish like salmon, cod, sardines. One way to remember many of the omega-3 rich fish is the mnemonic "SMASH+C," which stands for salmon, mackerel, anchovies, sardines, herring, and black cod. The oils in these fish are full of Docosahexanoic acid (DHA) and Eicosapentanoic acid (EPA)—fatty acids which are so effective in reducing inflammation. The vegan diet can be deficient in EPA and DHA, and some falsely believe that our body can convert ALA found in vegetables to EPA and DHA. In fact, humans only convert between 1% to 5% of vegetable ALA to the highly bioavailable EPA and DHA. EPA is cardioprotective and has many brain and anti-inflammatory benefits. DHA is neuroprotective as well as anti-inflammatory. We need both sources. I recommend increasing servings of omega-3 rich fish, preferably wild caught, to 4-5 servings a week to balance out the omega 6 ratio. Vegetarians would do well to incorporate fish oil supplements into their diet or consider an algae-based omega-3 supplement for strict vegetarians.

Whole Soy Foods

Soy can be an excellent source of plant protein. There are some caveats about soy. Soy in the US is primarily a GMO food. I recommend avoiding GMO foods because they are designed to withstand higher levels of pesticides without killing the plant. But why would you want to put that into your body? We already live in an increasingly toxic world without adding toxins to our foods. If you purchase a soy product, ensure the label reads "organic and non-GMO." In addition, soy is high in lectins, so the subset of the population with gastrointestinal auto-inflammatory conditions or autoimmune conditions may find that it exacerbates their autoimmune inflammation. Therefore, soy can be an excellent source of plant protein for many if it is organic, but it may not be a healthy choice for everyone, especially the 25 % of people in the world with an autoimmune syndrome. Sometimes people decide to adopt a "healthy" vegetarian diet after they are diagnosed with an autoimmune condition, thus increasing their intake of soy and gluten. If you feel amazing after you do so, you are on the right path. If you are experiencing ongoing struggles and fatigue, I recommend consulting a functional nutritionist to determine the correct choice of food combinations for you.

Superfood Group #5: Mushrooms

Mushrooms have polysaccharides that act as immune modulators. The polysaccharides in mushrooms improve the arm of the immune system that improves defenses against viruses. We call this arm the Th1 part of the of the immune system, and it is part of our cellular mediated immunity and tumor surveillance. This arm of immunity gets weaker as we age, which is why age is the number one risk factor for cancer development. Mushrooms are a great superfood to incorporate regularly into your diet. Asian mushrooms such as reishi and maitake seem to have the highest concentration of these beneficial polysaccharides, and there are several studies on their applications for various types of cancers. The caveat regarding mushrooms: always cook your mushrooms! Raw mushrooms, including the innocent white button mushrooms, contain toxins that are bad for your liver and are carcinogenic. White button mushrooms, for example, contain hydrazine, a compound used in rocket fuel by NASA. The next time you are at a salad bar, skip the section with raw mushrooms. The good news is that mushroom toxins are heat sensitive, so a light sauté makes the mushroom okay to eat. Cooking your mushrooms has a second benefit. Mushrooms have tough cell walls made of chitin and the beneficial polysaccharides are inside the cell walls, therefore cooking brings out a higher content of the beneficial polysaccharides, while eliminating any harmful substances. This is a perfect example of food alchemy. Cooking converts a potentially problematic food into super-food gold. I recommend mushroom supplements in many of my patients, and one of my favorites is cordyceps. The active ingredient, cordycepin, increases detoxification efficiency in the body by increasing production of superoxide dismutase, glutathione, and catalase in the body. Those are some of the major pathways of liver detoxification in the body.[15] Cordyceps is one of several mushrooms involved in clinical trials due to its anti-cancer properties.[16]

While cordyceps are not readily available to eat, shiitake mushrooms are available in most supermarkets and make a great weekly addition to your diet. Shiitake and maitake mushrooms have beta glucans that have also been studied for their anti-cancer and immune boosting properties.[17]

Animal Proteins

Moving up on the pyramid, you notice the boxes are getting smaller. Reduce intake of animal proteins to a few servings per week. Among animal proteins, I consider dairy and cured meats to the most toxic. Cured meats have added nitrites, sulfites as and other chemicals added to provide a long shelf life. Dairy is inflammatory to all mammals after weaning, and in humans this occurs after the age of 9-10, when children develop their set of adult teeth. We thus lose lactase production after our adult teeth grow. Because dairy cannot be digested, the intact molecules reach the small intestine, where they causes immune reactivity and inflammation. Not surprisingly, many of those I test have antibodies against dairy products. In addition, dairy contains casein, a neuroinflammatory protein which promotes intestinal inflammation and brain inflammation too. In patients with multiple sclerosis, casein causes damaging demyelination of neurons by cross-reactivity.[18] Lastly, in the United States most cow products are tainted with growth hormones and antibiotics. Gross! I would recommend eliminating or severely limiting this pro-inflammatory food, eating only the highest quality of organic and omega-3 eggs, while limiting processed meats, and choosing white meats like poultry preferentially.

Spices

Spices have many flavonoids and terpenes with a breadth of benefits, so I recommend making your food tasty and delicious. Turmeric is well known for its anti-inflammatory and anti-cancer properties. Cinnamon has metabolic benefits for lowering glucose, ginger promotes healthy digestion and is anti-inflammatory, etc. Many other spices, such as basil, cilantro, clove, each have unique health benefits. There are no restrictions on spices, unless you have a food intolerance to one of them, in which case you should avoid it. Salt is technically a seasoning, not a spice, and it can be pro-inflammatory in large quantities. It also raises blood pressure. I recommend limiting salt intake to approximately 2 grams daily while incorporating more potassium salts in your food and more spices.

Last, red wine and dark chocolate are healthy choices for your sweet tooth and your happy hour. Red wine contains a flavonoid called resveratrol in small quantities. Resveratrol has anti-inflammatory and longevity health benefits. Dark chocolate has flavanols with health benefits as well. In modest quantities, they are delightful and healthy choices to add to your diet. Caveat: For those with histamine intolerance, red wine may not be a good choice and may cause flushing, headaches, and increased acid production in the stomach.

Keep in mind that there are certain conditions, like autoimmune conditions, inflammatory bowel diseases like celiac disease, ulcerative colitis, and Crohn's disease, for which foods high in lectins are pro-inflammatory. A lectin is an anti-nutrient molecule that binds to certain carbohydrates, has hemagluttinin properties, and can cross-react with the immune system, making autoimmunity worse. This subset of patients will benefit from eliminating gluten, soy, dairy and certain foods from the nightshade and legume family. There is another subset of patients which have a histamine intolerance and benefit from a low histamine version of the Mediterranean diet, and yet others who cannot metabolize oxalates well and benefit from a low oxalate diet. If you think you have an auto-immune condition or have developed reactions and intolerances to certain foods that are normally considered healthy, I recommend that you get evaluated by a functional nutritionist to identify which modifications of the anti-inflammatory diet can be most beneficial for you.

The MIND diet has been recommended for COVID Long Haul in some literature. The Mediterranean-Dash Diet Intervention for Neuro-degenerative delay (MIND) diet is essentially the anti-inflammatory diet with restrictions on sodium to 2.3 grams daily while increasing potassium intake, and we have already discussed this. You can achieve this increase in potassium by cooking with a reduced salt product containing a 50/50 blend of sodium and potassium salts. Those who have developed POTS syndrome may need a higher sodium intake, and we will cover this in the POTS chapter. Eliminate or severely avoid the "evil triad" of foods listed below. Following the anti-inflammatory guidelines just described will give you the best evidence-based benefit of dietary approaches.

Avoid The 'Evil Triad' of Inflammatory Foods

If you are trying to lower inflammation, it is good idea to avoid ingesting inflammatory foods. The idea of eating more anti-inflammatory foods while hoping to resolve inflammation is counterproductive to your healing efforts. I recommend elimination of 3 universally inflammatory foods as you are trying to recover. The three inflammatory foods are refined carbohydrates/sugars, dairy products, and processed meats.

Sugars and Refined Carbohydrates

The evolution of our genetics adapted us to a diet that was only sporadically exposed to sugar in the form of fruits, which grew seasonally and were not available year-round. The system for adaptation of glucose loading is easily overwhelmed by the large volumes of sugars and refined carbohydrates that are nearly ubiquitous in the food industry, even if you are not someone that adds sugar to your food or consumes sweetened drinks regularly. Foreigners visiting the United States find it remarkable how sweetened everything is: from salad dressings to sauces, yogurts, breads, etc. Indeed, sixty percent of packaged food products in the supermarket isle have added sugar. After a while, newcomers lose their sensitivity to the sweet flavors but experience weight gain and weight-related health problems. We are not well adapted to the large number of sugars and refined carbohydrates in our diet, and frequent exposure leads to inflammation via mechanisms related to glycation-end-products—highly reactive and damaging radicals known to contribute to "inflammaging" of the body. The increased glycemic index of refined carbohydrates promotes insulin insensitivity, and increased secretion of insulin-like-growth factor-1 (IGF-1). IGF-1 is associated with activation of inflammatory pathways via Nuclear Factor Kappa Beta (NFKB-1) signaling, a highly inflammatory pathway.[19] NFKB is a protein associated with many functions in the body, and it is one of the main chemicals which activate the inflammatory pathways in the body by triggering production of cytokines. Cytokines are the molecular signals that activate pathways of inflammation, and high levels cause the famous "Cytokine storm" associated with COVID. Cancer cells also use NFKB for cell growth and to promote inflammation. IGF-1 has been implicated in invasive cancers as well as chronic inflammation.[20] Stevia and monk fruit are excellent substitutes for sugar and can be used liberally to sweeten your life.[21]

Dairy

Substitute your butter for organic clarified ghee and avoid or eliminate all other dairy products. The western diet is loaded with dairy products, yet dairy becomes inflammatory early on around the age of 9-10, when the gene that codes for lactase production gets turned off. Evolutionarily, all mammals, including humans, lose lactase production around the age of weaning. In humans, this happens around the age of 9-10 when children develop their adult teeth. When this happens, the body wisely decides that the child no longer needs mother's milk to survive. The lactose producing gene gets turned off, and we lose the ability to digest dairy. When undigested, large proteins enter the small intestine, they create immune reactivity against the food in the small intestine. This creates gastrointestinal inflammation, which subsequently becomes whole body inflammation. It is no surprise then that food antigen testing often reveals IgG-mediated antibodies against most dairy proteins. Keep in mind that IgG-mediated food antibodies are a "food sensitivity." This differs from a food "allergy" which is an IgE-mediated, life-threatening anaphylactic reaction that requires injection with an Epi-pen to control. Possibly because IgG-mediated food sensitivities are not life-threatening, people ignore this low-level chronic inflammation and immune activation for years, if not decades, until they get themselves into a non-healing state, react to many foods, and are unable to resolve their systemic inflammation. Dairy is even more problematic in the United States because of the ubiquitous contamination of dairy products with growth hormones and antibiotics in cow products. Growth hormones affect insulin signaling and are hormonal disruptors, and antibiotics are likely contributing to the rising rates of dysbiotic flora and IBS that I am seeing in clinic, as well as increased antibiotic resistance. Think about it, we are the only mammals on this earth that drink other mammal's milk well into old age. Does this seem natural to you? Would you think it is natural if instead it was your family dog drinking milk from a pregnant cow or one that is put into an artificially pregnant state by growth hormone injections?

Another problem dairy presents to the body is casein. Casein is the main protein in dairy, and it is both neuroinflammatory and inflammatory to the intestines. Many of my patients have cured their IBS symptoms simply by eliminating dairy from their diet. Casein has been implicated in demyelinating syndromes of the brain like multiple sclerosis and even autism.[22] It has been implicated in brain fog and increased phlegm production.[23] Milk casein has a protein called beta-casomorphin-7 that makes dairy highly addictive because it binds to opioid receptors, just like morphine does. People feel good at the expense of making themselves ill, not unlike other addictive behaviors. Not surprisingly, some people fight me tooth and nail on this recommendation. You may even be thinking right now "this part I am going to skip, but I will do everything else like the supplements." Ever try to convince someone with an addiction to kick a habit? You might feel you are talking to a stone wall. It sometimes takes someone the pit of desperation of severe illness and disability to motivate them to kick bad habits. Both dairy and sugar have addictive properties. Mouse studies giving mice the option to press a lever that feeds them sugar laced water versus cocaine found that the mice pressed the sugar water lever more often.[24] The anti-inflammatory diet is foundational to allowing the supplements to work, and I discourage anything other than your full commitment to the healing process.

Processed Meats

Deli meats and cured meats like salami, pastrami, smoked foods, and sausages have high amounts of additives like nitrates and sulfites, which give them their long and stable shelf life. These toxins overload our liver's ability to process the body's current toxin burden, thus slowing down the body's ability to move make meaningful movement towards resolution of inflammation. Think of it this way. Foods that have a long shelf life of 6 months to a year are likely highly processed. If yeast and bacteria refuse to consume the food, it is likely toxic, and you should refuse to eat this food as well.

When your body is inflamed, it is struggling to catch up to a metabolic debt, your organs are working overtime yet falling behind. Do you add to that debt while irrationally asking your body to heal? Or do you help your body do its work by stopping the behaviors that add to the inflammatory burden it already has?

As tantalizing as inflammatory foods are, I like to give this illustration. Imagine you just returned from an expensive international vacation you greatly enjoyed. On arriving home, your credit card debt is in the order of several thousand dollars to pay off the hotels, tours, dinners, and purchases made. Would this be a good time to go shopping for new clothes or a big-ticket purchase? A wiser choice would be to pay off your debt before any big retail purchases. So it is with the inflammatory debt in the body. Pay off your inflammatory debt before you ask your body to heal. Stay debt-free inflammation-wise to achieve sustained health.

The decision to fully commit to your healing, or derail it, is yours. Patients who want to take supplements only or pick which portion of the protocol they agree to follow–those are the patients that will fail to improve. You choose which side of progress you want to be on. Remember, nothing tastes as good as feeling healthy feels!

Case example: Georgia (name altered) is a 28-year-old woman who was referred to me by the UCSF pulmonary clinic for symptoms of Long Haul. She developed COVID in December 2021 during a family reunion. By the time I saw her eight months later, she continued to have exercise intolerance, fatigue, brain fog, and wheezing. In our first two visits, I ordered some labs and found she was deficient in vitamin D and had low ferritin levels. I recommended 5000 units of vitamin D3 and a well-tolerated form or iron called iron bis-glycinate that is not constipating. We went over the anti-inflammatory diet and the supplement regimen for Long Haul. Since she handled the food preparation for her family, she adopted the diet immediately by incorporating four to five servings of cruciferous vegetables, eating 3 servings of berries daily, and eating fatty fish three to four times weekly, while eliminating inflammatory foods like dairy and sugar. When I saw Georgia two months later in follow up, she reported feeling 80% better. She was back to exercising five days weekly and only used her inhaler sporadically. Other than vitamin D and the iron supplements, she had started none of the other supplements in the protocol, because she felt dramatically better after modifying her diet. In her case, simply eliminating dairy and fermented foods, which are high in histamine, correcting her low vitamin stores, while following the anti-inflammatory diet was enough to produce a dramatic improvement in a short period.

Now that you understand how to eat food as medicine, and some caveats to consider, we will discuss other sources of inflammation which can contribute to your Long-Haul symptoms.

Summary

- The anti-inflammatory diet is a plant-based diet with five servings of cruciferous vegetables, three servings of plant-based antioxidants coming from berries and pomegranate seeds, increased sources of omega-3 fatty acids, coming from both plants and fish, while reducing quantities of animal proteins. The anti-inflammatory diet limits salt to just over 2 grams daily and benefits from increasing potassium daily. You can cook with a 50/50 low salt product that combines the two salts to meet this requirement.
- Increase your fatty fish intake to three to four servings per week. Fish that are low in mercury and high in omega-3 fatty acids are the "SMASH + C" fish:
  - Salmon
  - Mackerel
  - Anchovies
  - Sardines
  - Herring
  - +Cod

- Use perilla oil instead of other nut-based cooking oils such as canola, for low heat cooking and as a finishing oil. Perilla oil contains 50-60 % ALA, a plant omega-3 fatty acid. Olive oil has lower quantities of omega-3 fatty acids (15%) and is also recommended. Other sources of omega-3 oils include flax seeds and hemp seeds. Substitute butter with organic clarified ghee butter for medium to high heat cooking.
- Humans on average only convert between 1-5% of plant omega-3 fats to the more bioavailable EPA/DHA omega-3's, so both types are needed. If you are vegetarian or vegan, you must supplement with fish oil or algae-based oils, which contain DHA and some EPA.
- Eating anti-inflammatory foods while avoiding "the evil triad" of pro-inflammatory foods like sugar, dairy and processed meats can have a benefit in lowering whole body inflammation.
- Diet is not a one-size-fits-all approach. Modifications to this diet could include elimination of high histamine foods, or elimination of lectins if you have autoimmune disease or inflammatory gastrointestinal disease.
- Consider referral to an integrative or functional nutritionist if you have a condition where you may have developed food sensitivities, if you have an autoimmune condition, have histamine intolerance, and may need personalized variations of this diet. There are several databases where you can find a specially trained dietitian: One is the dieticians from the Academy of Nutrition and Dietetics, the other is the Integrative and Functional Nutrition Academy.
  - integrativerd.org/home
  - www.ifnacademy.com

CHAPTER 4

Histamine Inflammation, Histamine Intolerance, and Mast Cell Activation

"The doctor of the future will give no medicine but will interest
his patient in the care of the human frame, in diet and in the
cause and prevention of disease."
Thomas Edison, 1903

A second driver of inflammation that is very important in producing fatigue symptoms is the pathway driven by histamine. Histamine-mediated inflammation can be seen in a broad array of diseases and symptoms and is a large enough problem that it deserves its own chapter. Histamine inflammation is especially prevalent in both COVID disease and in Long-COVID symptoms. A 2021 study[25] reported that famotidine, also known as Pepcid, had anti-viral activity against COVID infection because of its antihistamine properties, and due to the propensity of COVID infection to cause dysfunctional mast cell activation. Dr. Larry Afrin, an immunologist specializing in mast cell activation disease, has published numerous studies on the frequency of mast cell activation in patients with COVID Long-Haul symptoms.[26] Therefore, addressing histamine is key in recovery from Long Haul.

There is a spectrum of different histamine-mediated syndromes that I see in my chronic fatigue clinic: this range includes primary and secondary mast cell activation syndromes, histamine excess, histamine intolerance, and Th2 dominance, the latter three being most common. Th2 dominance means that your immune system is driven by a type of immune cell called a T-helper type 2 lymphocyte, or a Th2 cell. Th2 cells specialize in activating mast cells and in driving histamine-mediated inflammation. While primary mast cell activation is less common, secondary mast cell activation is seen in a significant subset of Long-Haul patients. Additionally, histamine excess due to a Th2-dominant immune system is very common, and the underlying driver of many of the symptoms that bring fatigued patients into my office. An immune system that is chronically activated in a histamine-mediated response is called a Th2 dominant immune system. While I sometimes diagnose mast cell activation or elevated plasma histamine, in the absence of these markers, Th2 dominance affects the great majority of patients. In those who have co-existent autoimmune disease, Th2-codominance is common as well.

Histamine is secreted by three types of white blood cells: mast cells, eosinophils, and basophils. A subset of patients recovering from COVID will experience symptoms due to mast cell activation or activation of one of the other histamine-producing cells. Histamine is a protective pathway that creates excess mucus and streams of bodily fluids. This can be an important defense against parasites, and it helps to remove allergens from nasal passages and airways. For example, if an allergen or a virus enters your nasal cavity, histamine activation causes sneezing and mucus production which flushes it out. If you develop a parasitic infection, diarrhea develops to flush it out, physically expelling the parasite from the intestinal tract. Vomiting can eject an infectious agent directly from the stomach. Histamine activates gastric acid secretion, thereby sterilizing our food. The histamine response is therefore a protective response of the immune system that has a "flushing out" utility. The signal that initiates this pathway is a cytokine called interleukin 4 (IL-4). IL-4 activates the Th2 commander cells, which in turn stimulate mast cells to secrete histamine granules. The Th2 cells secrete more interleukin 4 and some interleukin 13, activating histamine activity even more. Now we have a self-reinforcing loop of inflammation that can be hard to break. IL-4 activation of Th2 is illustrated in Figure 9, in the middle row.

Many of the symptoms of Long Haul, including gastritis, diarrhea, postural dizziness, insomnia, migraines, brain fog, shortness of breath and palpitations are mediated by excess histamine or mast cell activation. Figure 10 below, from a paper published by Dr. Afrin and colleagues, lists the manifestation of mast cell activation disease (MCAD). Symptoms of MCAD include fatigue, temperature changes, dry eyes, itchy red skin, throat pain, oral ulcers, lymph node swelling, cough or shortness of breath, fainting spells, palpitations, POTS, nausea, diarrhea, headaches, nerve pain, and hypersensitivity reactions. Notice how closely MCAD symptoms resemble those of CFS/ME and Long COVID.

Figure 9. T-HELPER-CELL DIFFERENTIATION

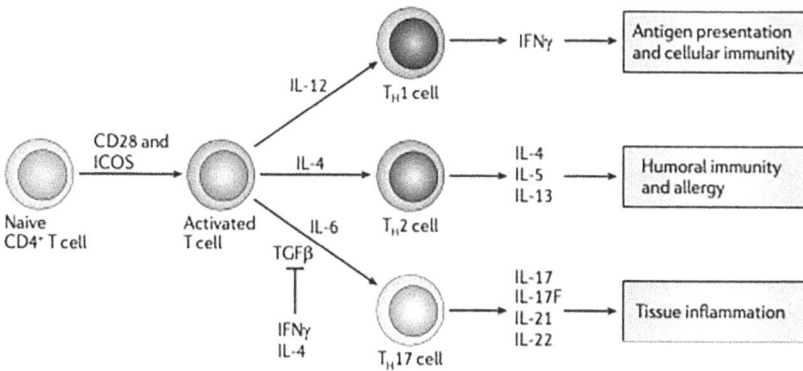

Naïve CD4$^+$ T cells, after activation by signalling through the T-cell receptor and co-stimulatory molecules such as CD28 and inductible T-cell co-stimulator (ICOS), can differentiate into one of three lineages of effector T helper (T_H) cells — T_H1, T_H2 or T_H17 cells. These cells produce different cytokines and have distinct immunoregulatory functions. Interferon-γ (IFNγ) produced by T_H1 cells is important in the regulation of antigen presentation and cellulary immunity. The T_H2-cell cytokines interleukin 4 (IL-4), IL-5 and IL-13 regulate B-cell responses and anti-parasite immunity and are crucial mediators of allergic diseases. T_H17 cells have been shown to express IL-17, IL-17F, IL-21 and IL-22 (and IL-26 in humans) and to regulate inflammatory responses. TGFβ, transforming growth factor-β. (Used with permission: *Natures Review Immunology*. ncbi.nlm.nih.gov/pmc/articles/PMC3703536/)[27]

Long-Haul patients often benefit from Pepcid/Famotidine, a selective histamine blocker, and other antihistamines like Benadryl/Diphenhydramine at bedtime. A 2020 article early in the pandemic found that adding famotidine 20 or 40 mg iv bid during acute COVID hospitalization significantly reduced risk of intubation in patients.[28] Famotidine was subsequently added to COVID hospital treatment protocols. Famotidine use was associated with improved clinical outcomes in hospitalized patients with COVID. Famotidine blocks a specific receptor called an H2 (histamine type 2) receptor. I have found that adding additional mast cell or antihistamine support in patients who were otherwise not responding to the anti-inflammatory treatment was the turning point in their recovery.

If you suspect you have histamine dominance or mast cell activation,

Figure 10. MANIFESTATION OF MAST CELL ACTIVATION DISEASE	
System	Potential manifestations of MCAD
Constitutional	Fatigue, subjective or objective hyperthermia and/or hypothermia, sweats, flushing, plethora or pallor, increased or decreased appetite, weight gain or loss, migratory pruritus, chemical/physical sensitivities (often "odd"), poor healing
Dermatologic/integument	Dermatographism, rashes/lesions of many sorts (migratory patchy macular erythema, telangiectasias, angiomata, xerosis, striae, warts, tags, folliculitis, ulcers, dyshydrotic eczema), angioedema, alopecia, onychodystrophy (e.g. brittle and/or longitudinally ridged nails)
Ophthalmologic	Irritated (often "dry") eyes, episodic difficulty focusing, lid tremor/tic (blepharospasm)
Otologic/osmic	Infectious or sterile otitis externa and/or media, hearing loss and/or tinnitus, dysosmia, coryza, post-nasal drip, congestion, epistaxis
Oral/oropharyngeal	Pain or irritation (sometimes "burning"), leukoplakia, ulcers, angioedema, dysgeusia, dental and/or periodontal inflammation/decay despite good personal and professional attention to dental hygiene
Lymphatic	Adenopathy (usually sub-pathologic and spontaneously waxing/waning in size, often migratory), adenitis, splenitis (typically only modest)
Pulmonary	Airway inflammation at any or all levels, cough, dyspnea (usually mild, episodic, "just can't catch a deep breath" despite normal pulmonary function tests), wheezing (usually quite mild), obstructive sleep apnea regardless of weight
Cardiovascular	Presyncope [co-diagnosis of postural orthostatic tachycardia syndrome (POTS) is common; full syncope is relatively rare], hypertension, blood pressure lability, palpitations (usually not correlating with electrocardiographic events), migratory edema, chest pain (usually non-anginal), atherosclerosis, odd heart failure (e.g. takotsubo), allergic angina (Kounis syndrome), vascular anomalies
Gastrointestinal	Dyspepsia, gastroesophageal reflux, nausea, vomiting (sometimes cyclical), diarrhea and/or constipation (often alternating), gastroparesis, angioedema, dysphagia (usually proximal), bloating/gas (usually post-prandial, often acute/subacute, sometimes to the appearance of full pregnancy), migratory abdominal pain from luminal or solid organ inflammation or distention, malabsorption; cholecystectomy is common, though often yielding normal pathology; ascites is rare
Genitourinary	Migratory luminal and solid organ inflammation ("urinary tract infection," often culture-negative, is commonly misdiagnosed instead of interstitial cystitis), chronic kidney disease, endometriosis, chronic back/flank/abdominal pain, infertility, decreased libido, vulvodynia, vaginitis (often misdiagnosed as infectious), painful and/or irregular dysmenorrhea, menorrhagia; miscarriages are common and occasionally signal an anti-phospholipid antibody syndrome possibly rooted in MCAS

System	Potential manifestations of MCAD
Musculoskeletal/ connective tissue	Migratory bone/joint/muscle pain (co-diagnosis of fibromyalgia is common), joint laxity/hypermobility [co-diagnosis of hypermobile Ehlers-Danlos syndrome (hEDS) is common], osteopenia/osteoporosis (osteosclerosis is seen but is rare), and other tissue growth/ development anomalies (i.e. dystrophisms, usually benign) such as cysts, fibrosis, vascular anomalies such as hemorrhoids, aneurysms, and arteriovenous malformations, occasionally even liquid or solid malignancies
Neurologic	Headache, sensory neuropathies (most commonly episode/migratory paresthesias in the distal extremities), episodic weakness (though proven motor neuropathy is rare), dysautonomias, seizure disorders, "pseudoseizures" (likely dysautonomic events), cognitive dysfunction (most commonly memory, concentration, and/or word-finding difficulties), dyssomnias (insomnia, frequent waking, hypersomnolence, non-restorative sleep, restless legs; less commonly or rarely: sleep apnea, sleepwalking, sleep talking, sleep paralysis, night terrors)
Psychiatric	Mood disturbances (e.g. depression, anger/irritability, mood lability), anxiety disorders (anxiety, panic, obsession-compulsion), attention deficit/hyperactivity; frank psychosis is rare
Endocrinologic/ metabolic	Abnormal electrolytes and liver function tests, hypo- or hyperthyroidism (often just sheer (but modest) lability of thyroid function), dyslipidemia, impaired glucose control (hyperglycemia, hypoglycemia, glycemic lability), hypo- or hyper-ferritinemia; nutritional deficiencies are often suspected but are relatively rare, more commonly micronutrient than general protein/calorie), delayed puberty; adrenal dysfunction is often suspected but rarely proven
Hematologic/ coagulopathic	Polycythemia or anemia [typically just mild, most commonly normocytic but sometimes macrocytic or microcytic; other causes (e.g. iron deficiency), whether consequent to MCAS or not, must be ruled out and addressed; note that "normal" erythropoietic parameters (a relative polycythemia?) may seem odd given the extent of chronic multisystem inflammation], leukocytosis or leukopenia (typically mild), monocytosis or eosinophilia or basophilia (typically modest, occasionally moderate or even robust), thrombocytosis or thrombocytopenia (typically mild), arterial and/or venous thromboembolic disease, otherwise inexplicable "easy" bruising/bleeding (co-diagnosis of mild type 1 von Willebrand disease is common, too); there usually is no histologic or molecular evidence of MC aberrancy in the marrow in MCAS, but sometimes a modest hypocellularity or mild myeloproliferative or myelodysplastic appearance is seen, insufficient for diagnosis of a myeloproliferative neoplasm or myelodysplastic syndrome, and genetic and flow cytometric analyses almost always are normal
Immunologic	Hypersensitivity reactions, increased risk for malignancy and autoimmunity, impaired healing, increased susceptibility to infection, increased or decreased levels of immunoglobulin of any isotype; monoclonal gammopathy of undetermined significance (MGUS) is occasionally seen

Few patients display all of these symptoms; most display subsets, and the heterogeneity of full clinical profiles among MCAD patients is extreme. Most symptoms are chronic and low-grade; some are persistent, but many are either episodic or waxing/waning. Alfrin, L.B. (2020.) Diagnosis of mast cell activation syndrome: a global "consensus-2" *Diagnosis*. doi.org/10.1515/dx-2020-0005 have your doctor check a plasma histamine and a tryptase level. There are other tests that can be ordered, but they are more difficult to get and may require an immunology consultation, such as 24-hour urine N-methylhista-mine (see table 2). I recommend avoiding any antihistamines for 72 hours before histamine testing. This includes medications like Claritin/loratadine, Allegra/fexofenadine, Benadryl/diphenhydramine, migraine medications like the triptans (for example: Sumatriptan), and acid blockers like Pepcid or the proton pump inhibitor class of drugs like Omeprazole. They are all histamine blockers, and they could adversely impact the accuracy of the test.

There are 3 main histamine receptors in of the body: histamine receptors 1,2 and 3. Different drugs block different histamine receptors throughout the body. If your histamine level is elevated, you can repeat the levels every 3 months as your symptoms recover on this program. If your tryptase level is elevated, you may have mast cell activation and would benefit from further evaluation by an immunologist. Dr. Afrin believes that up to 15-20% of the American population may be affected by some form of mast cell activation. Because the symptoms can affect multiple organs in strange ways, patients often spend years, if not decades, visiting various subspecialists without a correct diagnosis. Figure 11 lists the criteria for diagnosing mast cell activa-tion syndrome.[29]

Even if you do not have mast cell activation, you may well have a Th2 dominant immune system, or you may have histamine intolerance due to poor clearance by the liver. Do you suffer from allergies, asthma, post-nasal drip, migraines, IBS, or excessive stomach acid? These are all histamine driven processes and may be signs of histamine dominance. When we think of how common it is to have one or more of the above symptoms, it becomes evident that Th2 dominance is common in the population.

So, now we understand that most people are already Th2 dominant before they develop COVID. In addition, aging has been associated with decreased cell-mediated immunity, or the Th1 arm of immunity. Cell mediated immu-nity is our anti-viral and anti-tumor defense, also known as the Th1 immune pathway. As Th1 goes down, Th2 dominance goes up, so aging is associated with Th2 dominance too. Enter COVID, and the inflammation has escalated 1000-fold. You develop activated mast cells that are furiously pumping out histamine granules. Instead of allergies, you develop severe histamine side effects of brain fog, migraines and chronic cough or wheezing.

If you think you could have histamine intolerance due to either Th2 dom-inance or mast cell activation, consider modifying the anti-inflammatory diet to remove high histamine foods: all dairy, all fermented foods including yogurt, cheese, fermented alcohols like wine, beer, kimchi, and sauerkraut. Focus on fresh foods, as leftovers develop increased histamine levels with each passing day. For more information on the low histamine diet, refer to

Figure 11. CRITERIA FOR DIAGNOSING MAST CELL ACTIVATION

Criteria to define mast cell activation syndrome	WHO criteria to define systemic mastocytosis
Major criteria	**Major criterion**
1. Multifocal or disseminated dense infiltrates of mast cells in bone marrow biopsies and/or in sections of other extracutaneous organ(s) (e.g., gastrointestinal tract biopsies; CD117-, tryptase- and CD25-stained)	Multifocal dense infiltrates of mast cells (>15 mast cells in aggregates) in bone marrow biopsies and/or in sections of other extracutaneous organ(s) (CD117-, tryptase- and CD25-stained)
2. Unique constellation of clinical complaints as a result of a pathologically increased mast cell activity (mast cell mediator release syndrome)	
Minor criteria	**Minor criteria**
1. Mast cells in bone marrow or other extracutaneous organ(s) show an abnormal morphology (>25%) in bone marrow smears or in histologies	1. Mast cells in bone marrow or other extracutaneous organ(s) show an abnormal morphology (>25%) in bone marrow smears or in histologies
2. Mast cells in bone marrow express CD2 and/or CD25	2. Mast cells in bone marrow express CD2 and/or CD25
3. Detection of genetic changes in mast cells from blood, bone marrow or extracutaneous organs for which an impact on the state of activity of affected mast cells in terms of an increased activity has been proved.	3. c-kit mutation in tyrosine kinase at codon 816 in mast cells in extracutaneous organ(s)
4. Evidence of a pathologically increased release of mast cell mediators by determination of the content of	4. Serum total tryptase >20 ng/ml (does not apply in patients who have associated hematologic non-mast-cell lineage disease)
• tryptase in blood	
• N-methylhistamine in urine	
• heparin in blood	
• chromogranin A in blood	
• other mast cell-specific mediators (e.g., leukotrienes, prostaglandin D2)	

jhoonline.biomedcentral.com/articles/10.1186/1756-8722-4-10/tables/2

Appendix 2 on p. 122. If needed, you can consult an integrative nutritionist to help you set up a meal plan.

Histamine intolerance is one of the reasons why quercetin and vitamin C are essential in this protocol. Quercetin can stabilize mast cells, and vitamin C augments quercetin's effect.[30] Quercetin even has prophylactic properties against COVID.[31] In addition to quercetin and vitamin C, a few other botanicals have mast cell stabilizing properties as well: perilla, bromelain and astragalus. Perilla is a seed extract that can lower interleukin 4, the molecular signal that activates the entire histamine pathway. Perilla contains luteolin, apigenin, and rosemarinic acid as active constituents which give it antihistaminic properties.[32] Bromelain is a pineapple-stem-derived enzyme that has anti-fibrinolytic properties and mast cell stabilizing properties. Clot formation and fibrosis have been well documented in both COVID and in Long Haul, therefore this enzyme is very important in recovery.[33] Other anti-fibrinolytics such as serrapeptase and natto kinase are alternatives in someone with a bromelain intolerance due to pineapple allergies. Optionally, astragalus can be added to the histamine protocol. Astragalus lowers the cytokines interleukin 13 and GATA-3, thereby lowering overall inflammation in addition to histamine mediated inflammation. Astragalus is an adaptogen, meaning it helps to decrease the negative impacts of stress to the body. Astragalus has been studied in both cancer therapies and cancer-related fatigue.[34] By decreasing GATA-3, it provides a boost the anti-viral arm of the immune system and decreases Th2 dominance. Both Perilla and Astragalus have immune modulating activities, which means they can rebalance your immune system. Dosing for quercetin, perilla, vitamin C and astragalus are provided at the end of this chapter and in the supplements chapter. Lastly, if your blood histamine level is elevated, you can add S-Adenosyl-methionine (SAME) 200-800 mg daily to the mast cell protocol.[35] SAME promotes neutralization of active histamine by a process called methylation. After histamine is methylated, it becomes inert, it can no longer promote inflammation, and it is more easily eliminated by the body.[36] I do not recommend SAME if plasma histamine is normal, as SAME can cause methylation of other chemicals in the body with unknown consequences.

Drug therapies for mast cell activation include antihistamines such as hydroxyzine, diphenhydramine, compounded ketotifen, and mast cell stabilizers like cromolyn sodium. Some of these medications need insurance pre-authorization and may not be instantly available even with a prescription. Others, like ketotifen and cromolyn may only be available at compounding pharmacies. Because antihistamines block selected histamine receptors, they can lose effectiveness over time as the body adapts to the drug. The benefits of a botanical protocol include ready access, and unlike drugs, the COVID protocol includes carefully selected immune modulators that address the underlying inflammatory drive. Rather than losing effect, over time the effect of botanicals becomes more profound.

Supplements are not a panacea and have several disadvantages. Quality of supplements varies, and there are inefficiencies in bioavailability, making the dosing needed for effect to be larger. This results in a bigger pill burden. Supplements are not as fast acting as drugs, so the road to recovery looks more like a marathon, rather than a sprint. While supplements are generally deemed safe, there are some precautions that need to be taken to prevent side effects or interactions with certain drugs. I list some tips for supplements at the end of the supplement chapter. When it matters, I will list some supplements by name to prevent purchase of ineffective substitutes.

Commonly prescribed drugs for treating MCAS:
- Histamine 1 blockers—Hydroxyzine (Atarax), Doxepin (Silenor), Cyproheptadine (Periactin), Loratadine (Claritin), Fexofenadine (Allegra), Diphenhydramine (Benadryl), Ketotifen (Zaditen) and Cetirizine (Zyrtec, Reactine).
- Histamine 2 blockers—Famotidine (Pepcid, Pepcid AC), Cimetidine (Tagamet, Tagamet HB) and Ranitidine (Zantac). Famotidine is chosen most often because it has fewer drug interactions than Tagamet.
- Mast Cell Stabilizers—Cromolyn (Cromolyn Sodium, Gastrocom—oral form, Nasalcrom—nasal spray, Opticrom—eye drops, and there is a nebulized form and a cream can be made from a bottle of Nasalcrom and Eucerin or DMSO cream), Ketotifen (both a mast cell stabilizer and an H1 blocker) and Hydroxyurea (Hydrea).
- Mast Cell Inhibitors—Montelukast (Singulair), Zafirlukast (Accolate) and Zileuton (Zyflo). Pentosan (Elmiron) is used in the genitourinary tract for perineal pain and interstitial cystitis.
- Antibody neutralizers—Omalizumab (Xolair).
- Stimulants—Mixed salts amphetamine (Adderall XR), Methylphenidate (Ritalin) and Ephedrine (EpiPen provides an acute rescue injection when experiencing an anaphylactic episode).

The symptoms experienced by Long-COVID patients are strikingly like symptoms experienced by people diagnosed with chronic fatigue syndrome/myalgic encephalitis (CFS/ME). A research article examining several inflammatory markers (cytokines) in people diagnosed with CFS/ME found that subjects with CFS/ME had several inflammatory pathways activated all at once, including high levels of 13 proinflammatory cytokines, compared with healthy subjects. Not surprisingly, studies of people with Long-COVID found a similar pattern with many of the same inflammatory markers. Interestingly, the patterns of inflammation varied from one person to another, much like an inflammatory fingerprint. Yet both studies showed high Interleukin 4 and Interleukin 13 as a common pattern—the markers of mast cell activation. TGF-β was elevated in CFS patients, and this marker was sensitive for tracking severity of fatigue symptoms. The higher the TGF-β, the more debilitating the fatigue. TGF-β beta is a bone marrow signaling protein which lowers inflammation, but it does so at the expense of causing immune suppression and fibrosis of organs. TGF-β can be lowered by increasing antioxidant reserves, which I will discuss in the toxins chapter. Notably, both CFS/ME sufferers and Long Haulers had elevated markers for mast cell activation, namely IL-4 and IL-13.

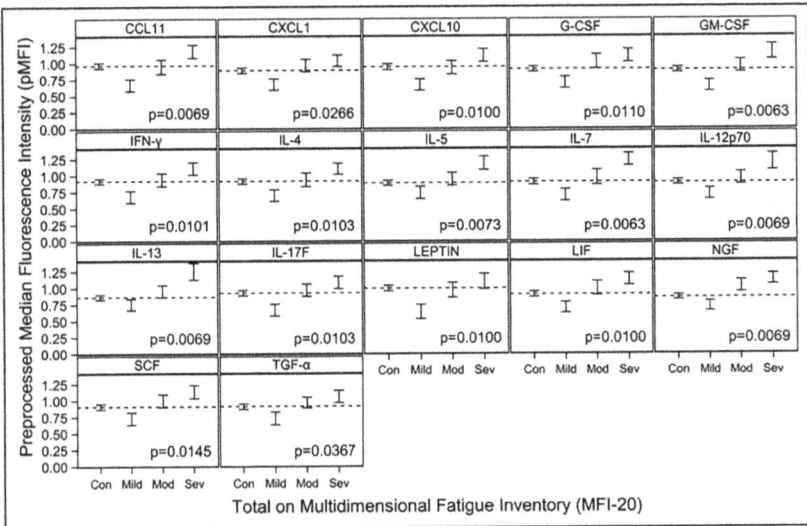

Figure 12. INFLAMMATORY MARKERS FOUND IN CFS/ME

Mean cytokine levels with statistically significant linear trends in ME/CFS patients grouped by mild, moderate (Mod), and severe (Sev) disease compared with healthy controls (Con). Mean pMFI ± 1 SE are shown as vertical brackets for each cytokine. *P* values shown are for the significance of the linear trend. Only statistically significant linear trends adjusted for multiple comparisons ($P < 0.05$) are shown. All results shown in this figure were also adjusted for age, sex, race, and nonspecific binding. The dotted horizontal line within each cytokine panel represents the average value for healthy controls.

Montoya, J.G. (2017). Cytokine signature associated with disease severity in chronic fatigue syndrome patients. Adapted with permission.

Figure 13. INFLAMMATORY PATTERNS FOUND IN LONG-HAUL PATIENTS

TNF-ALPHA	52.3	HIGH	pg/mL	< 11.0
IL-4	102.0	HIGH	pg/mL	< 6.2
IL-13	31.5	HIGH	pg/mL	< 6.1
IL-2	10.0	HIGH	pg/mL	< 7.0
IL-6	13.5	HIGH	pg/mL	< 3.0
IL-10	2.4	HIGH	pg/mL	< 1.0
IFN-GAMMA	14.6	HIGH	pg/mL	< 3.5
LONG HAULER INDEX	0.78	HIGH	INDEX	< 0.71

Radiance Diagnostics Cytokine panel: Inflammatory patterns found in a typical patient with Long Haul: Elevated IL-4 and IL-13 are markers for mast cell activation and histamine mediated inflammation. IL-6 is associated with classic inflammation

Lastly, let's talk about clearance of histamine from the body. There are patients who have symptoms identical to mast cell activation, but instead their symptoms are due to histamine buildup in the body. How does this happen? Histamine gets broken down in the liver by an enzyme called Aldehyde Dehydrogenase, or ALDH, while Diamine Oxidase (DAO) breaks down histamine in the intestine. ALDH is an enzyme is involved in the breakdown of both alcohol and histamine.[37] ALDH needs four cofactors to function: Iron, vitamin B2, B3, and Molybdenum. For a long time, I wondered why there are more women in my clinic with chronic fatigue, migraines, and brain fog. When I started checking plasma histamine levels, I found many patients had elevated histamine levels. I then started checking vitamin B2 and ferritin, a good marker of total body iron. Many of these levels were low as well. Ferritin is a more sensitive marker for iron deficiency than a serum iron level, since it measures total body iron stores. Low ferritin stores are a double plague: not only are you inflamed because your liver cannot break down histamine, but you also suffer from decreased oxygen-carrying capacity and exercise intolerance because you shift into anaerobic metabolism with even with mild exercise. This causes post-exertional malaise and muscle aches. Many women with exercise intolerance and fatigue get incorrectly diagnosed with fibromyalgia, yet their symptoms dramatically improve when I correct their iron and low vitamin B2 levels. Low oxygen carrying capacity drives the body to secrete a chemical called HIF-1 alpha (hypoxia inducible factor-1 alpha), which stimulates more inflammation before it signals the bone marrow to produce more red blood cells—if there is enough iron to do so. Living with low ferritin stores is therefore a bit like living in high altitude, except you never adapt. Instead, you get sicker and sicker. Ferritin can be falsely elevated during an acute infection, so I do not recommend getting it checked if you are currently fighting an infection.

Many women live their lives with borderline low ferritin or even mild anemia, and it is largely ignored by the medical community because doctors are taught that iron deficiency is normal in women, and it does not need any action. However, when women become disabled by their chronic fatigue, migraines, and brain fog, and can no longer sustain a job, they are incorrectly diagnosed with fibromyalgia or made to feel "it is all in their head." Current medical practice neglects to understand and address the several inflammatory pathways activated by iron deficiency, as medical protocols are largely driven by male-dominated research that increases health disparities among minorities and women.[38] Low ferritin levels below 30 ng/mL alone can cause a fibromyalgia-like syndrome: exercise intolerance due to chronic low-grade hypoxia, chronic fatigue, and chronic muscle aches, since even walking around the house will cause a shift into anaerobic metabolism. Rheumatology guidelines should be updated to reflect this—a diagnosis of fibromyalgia should only be made after conditions such as ferritin deficiency and vitamin D deficiency have been properly addressed. I can't tell you how many fibromyalgia, restless legs, and mast cell activation symptoms simply disappeared once the ferritin levels were optimized to reach a level of 100 ng/ml. It would avoid a great deal of the confusion and the stigma this diagnosis carries. The good news is that the medical establishment recognizes the bias in research and efforts are underway to address it in future research. For now, we are left with standards of care that routinely ignore these simple women's health needs.

While low iron stores contribute to fatigue and symptoms of mast cell activation, high iron stores are equally problematic, as they have been linked to cardiovascular disease and cancer risk. The health risks from high iron are due to its ability to easily oxidize. You see this when an iron table or chair gets rusty. Excessive iron similarly generates oxidative free radicals in the body, subjecting cells to damage. This oxidation process is called the Fenton reaction. Therefore, iron levels should be followed closely when supplementing, to avoid overcorrection. I like to give patients glutathione as I correct their iron, because glutathione is an antioxidant that neutralizes free radicals to produce water, as you can see in the chemical reaction below. The goal ferritin level should be no higher than 100 ng/mL, which is the goldilocks zone, not too low, not too high. Most women I see with fatigue have ferritin levels in the 10-30 ng/mL range, with 12 being the cutoff for normal. I consider any ferritin level below 100 ng/mL to be suboptimal, and any level below 60 ng/ml as likely contributing to symptoms of fatigue.

Figure 14. FENTON REACTION AND GLUTATHIONE

Fenton reaction
(Catalyzed by iron or copper)

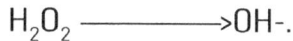

$$H_2O_2 \longrightarrow OH\text{-}.$$

Glutathione
(GSH)

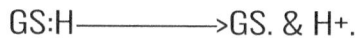

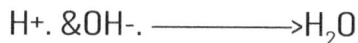

$$GS{:}H \longrightarrow GS. \ \& \ H\text{+}.$$

$$H\text{+}. \ \& OH\text{-}. \longrightarrow H_2O$$

B2: Vitamin B2 (Riboflavin) is the second nutrient needed by the ALDH enzyme to break down histamine. When you review the medical literature, B2 deficiency is categorized as a 'rare' deficiency. In fact, most B complexes do not contain B2, since riboflavin deficiency is supposed to be uncommon. Yet riboflavin is key in supporting ALDH breakdown of histamine, and it is also important in recirculation of glutathione, the major antioxidant produced by the liver. I ordered a B2 level for the first time in my career 16 years into medical practice, when I learned about the link between high histamine and iron/B2/B3 deficiency. Once I started seeing the high histamine and/or tryptase levels in patients, I embarked on the detective work to look at the entire chain in this cellular pathway from beginning to end with astounding results. I now diagnose B2 in the subset of patients referred to my clinic, in addition to low ferritin pretty much daily. Is B2 deficiency rare, or simply underdiagnosed?[39] I believe ferritin and B2 deficiency is common in patients who suffer from chronic fatigue, but we need further research on the matter.

If you think you have histamine excess adding to your inflammation, I recommend having histamine, B2, B3, and ferritin levels checked, and following a low histamine diet. In the supplements chapter of this book, we will go over the supplements for lowering histamine as part of the Long-

Haul protocol. They include quercetin, bromelain, perilla, vitamin C, and astragalus.

Low Histamine Diet

Reduce or avoid the following:

- Alcohol, especially fermented alcohols: wine, champagne, beer
- Smoked and cured meats
- Seafood
- Pickled foods
- Fermented foods, including yogurt and cheese
- Leftovers
- Canned fish or meat
- Berries, especially strawberries
- Nightshades, including tomatoes and potatoes
- Preservatives
- Vinegar

You can see how seafood is emphasized in the anti-inflammatory diet but can be problematic due to its higher histamine content. Therefore, you may want to substitute fish oil and follow the low histamine diet for the first 2-3 months after starting the protocol. Once you begin to lower histamine in your body, you will be able to start tolerating these healthy foods and can reintroduce them slowly back into your diet. Some people addition-ally benefit from trying a digestive aid that breaks down histamine in food, called diamine oxidase, or DAO.[40] DAO supplements can be found in most supplement stores and online retailers and could allow you to enjoy these healthy foods.[41]

Resources for low histamine diet, recipes and meal planning can be found in the Appendix. You can find a pdf of the low histamine diet compiled by a Swiss research group—histaminintoleranz.ch/downloads/SIGHI-Leaflet_HistamineEliminationDiet.pdf

Summary

- Histamine-mediated inflammation is a major pathway of inflammation in both CFS/ME and Long COVID. It can range from histamine intolerance, Th2 dominance, to mast cell activation disease. According to Dr. Afrin, a specialist in mast cell activation, it may be more common than we think, affecting up to 15-20% of the North American population.
- COVID seems to promote unhealthy mast cell activation and therefore famotidine, and other classes of antihistamine drug therapies have been effective at improving outcomes in acute COVID infections. Mast cell activation seems to persist in a significant number of Long Haulers.
- If you suspect you have excess histamine or mast cell activation, consider following a low histamine diet for 2-3 months as you work on lowering histamine-mediated inflammation. You will find you tolerate these foods better in the future once inflammation is lower. Some people find DAO enzymes with food to be helpful in this stage.
- Ask your doctor to check a baseline histamine and tryptase level, along with ferritin, B2, B3 levels to see if you have a correctible deficiency.
- Supplements which treat mast cell activation and histamine excess include quercetin, bromelain, vitamin C, perilla (QBC + perilla), and astragalus. Bromelain has additional anti-fibrinolytic properties and is important in Long-COVID symptoms.

Mast Cell Protocol
- Perilla 150 mg twice daily (Pure Encapsulations or Metagenics Perimine)
- Quercetin 1500 mg daily in divided doses, either with food or in liposomal form
- Bromelain 1200-2400 units twice in between meals
- Vitamin C 1000 mg in divided doses

- Optional: Astragalus 1000-3000 mg daily in divided doses
- Optional: SAME 200-400 mg twice daily if plasma histamine elevated. (Caution in patients with bipolar disorder or mania)
- Optional: DAO enzymes with food

- Breaking down histamine: The liver needs iron, B2, B3 and Molybdenum to clear histamine though an enzyme called ALDH. Borderline ferritin is reflective of low iron stores and is commonly seen in chronic fatigue, low B2 and low B3 are common, and these deficiencies should be corrected in patients experiencing fatigue. Molybdenum deficiencies are less common. Iron deficiency is common, it can mimic symptoms of fibromyalgia

and should be corrected before this diagnosis is made.
- Correct any ferritin below 100 ng/ml. Fatigue can set in when ferritin is below 60 ng/ml. When correcting low iron stores, it is important to consider increasing antioxidant support to prevent the Fenton reaction, a temporary increase in oxidative free radicals in the body due to the oxidation of iron. This can be accomplished with use of antioxidants such as liposomal glutathione. Antioxidants are covered in the next chapter.

CHAPTER 5

Toxin Overload

"The elimination of toxins awakens the capacity for renewal."
Deepak Chopra

We have so far covered two major inflammatory pathways which cause fatigue: classic and histamine-mediated inflammation. Remember the three other buckets of fatigue? An important driver of symptoms is too many circulating toxins. Infection and its resolution are processes which generate many toxins. Cellular death and microbial death increase the toxic burden on the body, which must be cleared by the liver and kidneys.

Think of a city after a battle—there is a lot of rubble that needs to be

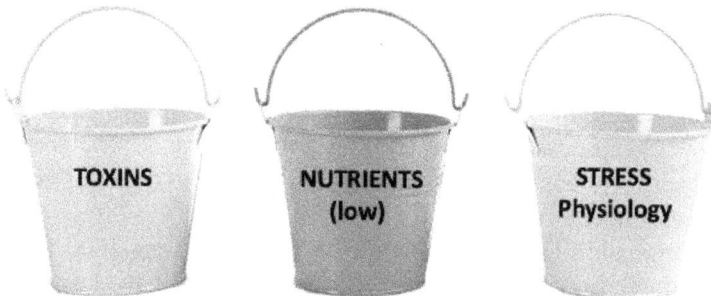

Figure 15: TOO MANY TOXINS

TOXINS

NUTRIENTS
(low)

STRESS
Physiology

cleaned up before the city can be rebuilt. Not surprisingly, patients who have high amounts of chronic pathogen burden, such as tuberculosis, Lyme, and chronically high burden of the EBV virus (the virus responsible for mononucleosis), suffer from fatigue. Inflammation itself can also cause increased cellular death, contributing to toxic burden even more. We now have a self-reinforcing mechanism: toxins create inflammation, and inflammation creates more toxins. To fully resolve inflammation, it is essential to increase toxin clearance from the body while you are working to decrease inflammation. I think of antioxidants and anti-inflammatories as the right and left hand of inflammation resolution.

To promote viral proliferation, viruses such as COVID-19 alter TGF-β signaling through a variety of mechanisms.[42] Besides eating a diet rich in antioxidants and taking vitamin C, it is good to aid the liver in its role of detoxifying the body. One of the main pathways of detoxification in our body is the glutathione peroxidase system. Glutathione is a tri-peptide molecule made by the liver from the precursor N-acetylcysteine (NAC). Glutathione binds electrons in reactive oxygen species and neutralizes them, making them easier to eliminate in the urine as water. The chemical reaction is below.

Figure 16. GLUTATHIONE DETOXIFICATION

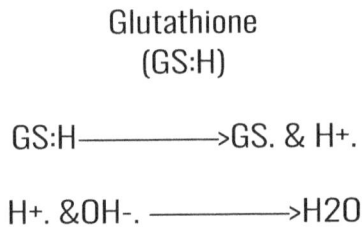

Glutathione
(GS:H)

$$GS:H \longrightarrow GS. \ \& \ H+.$$

$$H+. \ \& OH-. \longrightarrow H2O$$

To support the liver, you can take either the precursor NAC or liposomal glutathione. Your liver converts NAC to glutathione via an enzyme called glutathione-transferase, coded by a gene GTSP1. Some people have low levels of the enzyme because of allelic variations in this gene. Those people may find themselves easily reacting to antibiotics and may have environmental sensitivities because of an impaired ability to detoxify chemicals in their environment.

I recommend high doses of NAC, between 1500 mg-2700 mg daily in divided doses for CFS or Long COVID. In some who have low glutathione transferase enzyme activity because of a genetic (GSTP1) variant, they may be less able to convert NAC to the final molecule of glutathione. Those may find more benefit from taking liposomal glutathione, which is the final, bio-available version of this antioxidant. Glutathione is a fat-soluble molecule; therefore, it is poorly absorbed unless it is taken in the liposomal form, or if taken with food. Because NAC can be taken with or without food, it is the easier antioxidant to take. I recommend starting with NAC first, and if you see no benefits, consider switching to liposomal glutathione.

Besides increasing cellular stores of glutathione, consider the co-factors that your liver needs to make glutathione. Selenium and vitamin C are both needed. Riboflavin, or vitamin B2, supports the recycling of glutathione, so it is crucial for increasing antioxidant reserves, and we already discussed its role in histamine breakdown. You can get adequate daily selenium by eating two Brazil nuts daily, since Brazil nuts have the highest selenium content of all foods. A small packet will last you for several months if stored in the refrigerator.

It is important to reduce exposure to toxins. Eat organic foods when possible and avoid foods packaged with preservatives. Drink the best sources of water. Purified water from a reverse osmosis filter is the only way to remove certain organic acids and toxins which are found in the water. If you live in an area where the quality of your water may be compromised, or in an older house that may have rusted pipes, I recommend this form of water filtration. The initial investment will pay off as you save on the purchase of water bottles. You can also feel good about the reduction of plastic waste in your household. Using air purifiers in the home is important if you live in an urban area or have pollutants nearby. Avoiding food additives such as nitrites, sulfites and monosodium glutamate is important. Even perfumes and fragrances must be detoxified by the liver and use up precious reserves of glutathione. If you have developed sensitivity to fragrances, or other chemical sensitivities, this could be a sign that you are deficient in glutathione.

We live in an increasingly toxin-riddled world. The EPA has started acting against "forever chemicals" found in the water supply called perfluorooctanoic acid (PFOA).[43] The CDC has tested and found detectable levels of this chemical in almost everyone since 1999.

In a more recent 2022 report, the CDC found that phthalates and glyphosates are universally found in human urine.[44] Glyphosates come from the agricultural sprays such as Roundup. They have been linked to the adversely affecting the human microbiome and potentially giving rise to inflammatory gastrointestinal disorders due to increased intestinal permeability, known as leaky gut syndrome. Glyphosates function as endocrine disruptors and negatively affect your hormonal balance, too. Therefore, detoxification is more important today than in was in our grandparent's time.

Be aware of the "Dirty dozen" foods, which are higher in agricultural toxins. Plan to buy those foods from organic sources if possible. Generally, these are foods with thin skins like berries and celery. Fortunately, not all foods need to be organic. The foods known as the "Clean 15" are less problematic. I like to think of "The Clean 15" foods as those which have thick peels which we discard, like onions and avocados. The thick peels act as a barrier against agricultural sprays. If you would like to download and print the "dirty dozen" please see the appendix at the end of this book.

Figure 17: CLEAN FIFTEEN and DIRTY DOZEN

Clean Fifteen (Okay to buy conventional)	Dirty Dozen (Buy organic, if possible)
1. Avocados	1. Strawberries
2. Sweet corn	2. Kale, Collards, Mustard greens
3. Pineapple	3. Spinach
4. Onions	4. Nectarines
5. Papaya	5. Apples
6. Sweet peas (frozen)	6. Grapes
7. Eggplant	7. Cherries
8. Asparagus	8. Peaches
9. Broccoli	9. Pears
10. Cabbage	10. Peppers
11. Kiwi	11. Celery
12. Cauliflower	12. Tomatoes
13. Mushrooms	
14. Honeydew	
15. Cantaloupe	

osher.ucsf.edu/putting-nutrition-practice-tips-making-dietary-changes. Used with permission.

Remember the study which looked at the inflammatory cytokine signature in CFS/ME? The marker that stood out the most was transforming growth factor beta (TGF-β).[45] The higher the TGF-β level, the more disabling were the symptoms of CFS including cognitive dysfunction. TGF-β is often elevated in both chronic illness and in chronic fatigue. It has been associated with synchronization of several cellular signaling mechanisms including CLOCK genes implicated in loss of circadian rhythms, well known in CFS.[46] An unregulated TGF-β response has been documented in severe COVID-19 infection as well.[47] Increasing glutathione levels intracellularly lowers TGF-β and is why adding antioxidants to your diet while reducing toxin exposure is key to turning around symptoms of inflammation and fatigue.[48] Decreased glutathione levels have been linked to increased fibrosis, and a study showed that glutathione was helpful in preventing the progression of fibrosis. Therefore, in those who have developed pulmonary fibrosis or other organ fibrosis after recovering from COVID, replenishing glutathione stores can be a good idea.[49]

Finally, it is important to evaluate your living situation for environmental and mental toxins. If you live in a toxic house that is contaminated with mold, start planning your move today. If your workplace has become toxic, begin planning your next career move. Get rid of toxic friends—it is better to have fewer friends that are supportive of your dreams and aspirations. If your family is toxic, you may walk away. Some of these changes may take careful planning and time, especially if financial ties are present. But it is not only possible, it is necessary.

Glutathione is normally used prior to urine assays for black mold, as it draws mold out of the body into the urine. If you have severe "die off" reactions when you start even a low dose of glutathione, consider having your home evaluated for black mold, and consider evaluation by a practitioner trained to treat mold toxicity.

If you would like to enroll in clinical studies for COVID Long Haul, there are many universities that are closely following this syndrome and studying biomarkers of the disease. UCSF has a LIINK study (Long-term Impact of Infection with Novel Coronavirus) available on the clinical trials website, (clinicaltrials.ucsf.edu), and they are currently enrolling patients. It would be helpful if newer studies incorporated TGF-β analysis in cytokine analysis of Long-COVID patients, given the similarities with CFS and the high level of organ fibrosis seen COVID patients.

Summary

- Toxin overload is an important bucket to address in fatigue.
- Toxin burden can promote inflammation if not addressed. Think of anti-inflammatory agents and antioxidants as the right and left hand of decreasing inflammation.

- Infections cause an increased toxic burden on the body. Patients with high pathogen burden are more likely to exhaust their antioxidant reserves.
- Glutathione is produced by the liver from the precursor NAC, and it is one of the major detoxification agents in the body. You can support the liver by taking either NAC or liposomal glutathione.
- Glutathione decreases TGF-β, a marker elevated in CFS. High TGF-β is seen in fibrotic conditions too. Therefore, glutathione can be helpful in fibrotic conditions such as post COVID lung fibrosis.
- Reduce toxins in your environment by knowing the "dirty dozen" foods. Those foods are best bought organic. Drink filtered water from a reverse osmosis filter and reduce the intake of processed foods.
- Evaluate your living situation and consider removing yourself from toxic environments, even if it takes some advanced planning.

CHAPTER 6

The GI-Immune Axis

"The gut-or 'second brain' contains about 100 million neurons
that influence our emotions. Turns out 'listen to our gut'
is pretty good advice after all."
Dustin Lien

"All disease begins in the gut."
Hippocrates (460-370 B.C)

The next two co-conspirators in increased inflammatory drive are gastrointestinal inflammation and immune dysfunction. Your microbiome contains ten times more bacteria than there are cells in your body. Your intestines contain 80% of your lymphoid immune system through the GALT, or gut-associated lymphoid tissue. And the gut is hard-wired into the brain via a vast connection of shared neurons. In fact, the gut is often referred to as the "second brain" in the body, as it is the largest collection of neurons outside of the brain. It is no surprise then that extra-intestinal manifestations of poor gut health can impact brain function, immune function, and systemic inflammation. The importance of the human microbiome is gaining increasing traction in the medical world as more data emerges on its importance in maintaining good health.[50] At UCSF, a brand-new building built in 2020 was dedicated to microbiome research.

The gut-associated lymphoid tissue (GALT) contains about 80% of your antibody-producing cells, called lymphocytes. It is not surprising that unhealthy gut flora is often seen in patients with autoimmunity and fatigue, besides increased intestinal permeability, known as "leaky gut."

61

In fatigued patients, there is often a triangle of immune-gut-brain inflammation. It's no wonder then that an inflamed gut can cause brain and immune dysfunction, causing the symptoms of CFS of brain fog, fatigue, food sensitivities, and increased susceptibility to viral reactivation or new infections!

COVID infection can disrupt the microbiome ecosystem to promote gastrointestinal inflammation. There is emerging evidence of bacterial translocation from the intestines and development of leaky gut, that can contribute to development of Long COVID. When this breakdown of intestinal barriers is not addressed, over time, the increased permeability can lead to the development of food sensitivities, diagnosed by the presence of Ig-G antibodies against specific foods. This differs from food allergies, which are diagnosed by Ig-E antibodies. I have been impressed at how much easier it is to address autoimmune conditions and fatigue symptoms once the gastrointestinal inflammation has been properly addressed. It sets the foundation for the brain and immune system to work properly again.

If you have symptoms of indigestion, gas and bloating, or diarrhea, food sensitivities, you may have experienced a shift in your microbiome and may have developed inflammatory bowel syndrome (IBS) The global burden of IBS is currently estimated to affect 11% of the world population.[51] So, IBS is relatively common. In the chronically fatigued patients I see, IBS is present in most, with rare exceptions. Diagnostics for IBS include breath testing for bacterial overgrowth and microbiome testing. Currently, few gastrointestinal doctors test for and treat IBS. If your GI doctor does not perform breath testing or microbiome testing, you may seek a medical practitioner with integrative or functional training. You can find a functional medicine practitioner in the Society of Functional Medicine (ifm. org/find-a-practitioner/).

In my clinical experience, recognizing and addressing poor gut health if often pivotal in turning fatigue symptoms that were previously refractory to all other treatments. Therefore, I have a low threshold for ordering gastrointestinal and microbiome testing in fatigued patients who report any changes in digestive health. In the case of Hippocrates, one could rephrase his saying to "all disease begins in the *(leaky)* gut."

Therefore, if new or worsening gastrointestinal symptoms are part of your Long-COVID syndrome, I encourage you to get evaluated and "listen to your gut."

Addressing autoimmunity, immune dysfunction, and gut health probably beyond the scope of this book. Each topic could easily deserve a book of its own. I will keep my recommendations brief as they apply to Long Haul and CFS patients. Patients with autoimmune conditions frequently have concurrent gastrointestinal dysbiosis, IBS, food sensitivities, increased intestinal permeability, and cross-reactivity to lectin-containing foods. Lectin-containing foods include gluten, soy, and many foods from the nightshade and legume family. For the 25% of people in the world living with an autoimmune disease, dietary lectins are their kryptonite—it completely robs them of their strength. Worse, by an immune process called cross-reactivity, they react with the immune cells producing self-antibodies, further stimulating the autoimmune process and organ damage. If there is autoimmunity, I recommend starting with a strict gluten-free, soy-free, dairy-free diet, eliminating kidney beans, and pressure cooking all other beans. You may want to try a two-month elimination of legumes and nightshades, then reintroducing the legumes or nightshades one at a time each week to see which of those foods cause fatigue or digestive symptoms. You would do well to request testing for Celiac disease soon after starting a gluten-free diet. TTG antibodies are present in Celiac disease, and Gliadin antibodies are markers of non-celiac gluten reactivity, which manifests the same as Celiac disease. This blood test is only sensitive while consuming a gluten-rich diet, as the markers normalize in approximately 3 months after starting a gluten-free diet. Many who benefit from eliminating gluten and remain gluten-free miss the narrow 3-month window to test for Celiac disease or gliadin sensitivity. If you experience a benefit with this dietary modification, aim to get tested for these markers as soon as possible. If you have known or suspected autoimmunity, you may consider a consultation with a functional nutritionist because you may need to modify the anti-inflammatory diet in several important ways.

Having a pre-existing autoimmune condition is a risk factor for the development of Long COVID. It's also possible to have a new flare of your autoimmune condition after recovery from COVID, even if your condition was previously well controlled. COVID can kick the hornet's nest of any pre-existing inflammation in the body. What I normally see is that CRP, the indirect marker for interleukin 6, or classic inflammation, goes up during COVID infection. As the infection clears and CRP normalizes, sometimes auto-antibody levels such as the anti-nuclear antibody (ANA) will rise within a month after recovery, and an autoimmune flare may manifest. There is speculation that COVID can cause brand new autoimmunity as well. This would not be surprising, since high sustained inflammation can drive the immune system to act in a dysfunctional way. Going back to the image with three main pathways of inflammation, the bottom arm of "classic" inflammation is driven by IL-6, and it activates a Th17 cell. Activated Th17 cells are implicated in tissue damage and development of autoimmunity (See Figure 18).

Figure 18. T-HELPER-CELL DIFFERENTIATION

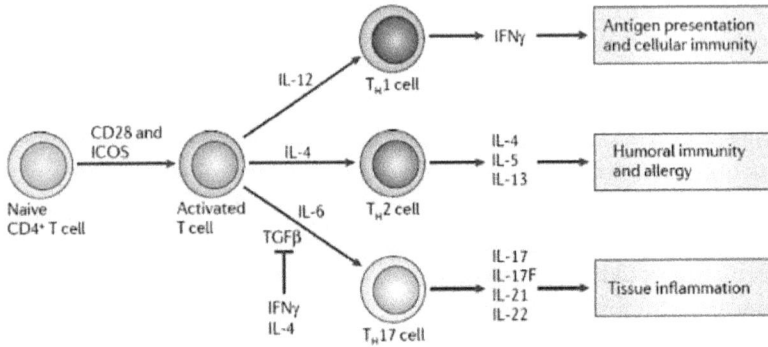

Naïve CD4$^+$ T cells, after activation by signalling through the T-cell receptor and co-stimulatory molecules such as CD28 and inductible T-cell co-stimulator (ICOS), can differentiate into one of three lineages of effector T helper (T$_H$) cells — T$_H$1, T$_H$2 or T$_H$17 cells. These cells produce different cytokines and have distinct immunoregulatory functions. Interferon-γ (IFNγ) produced by T$_H$1 cells is important in the regulation of antigen presentation and cellulary immunity. The T$_H$2-cell cytokines interleukin 4 (IL-4), IL-5 and IL-13 regulate B-cell responses and anti-parasite immunity and are crucial mediators of allergic diseases. T$_H$17 cells have been shown to express IL-17, IL-17F, IL-21 and IL-22 (and IL-26 in humans) and to regulate inflammatory responses. TGFβ, transforming growth factor-β. (Used with permission: *Natures Review Immunology*. ncbi.nlm.nih.gov/pmc/articles/PMC3703536/)

Probably the most common autoimmune condition I see in clinic is Hashimoto's hypothyroidism. Hashimoto's is an autoimmune condition and the most common cause of hypothyroidism. Many who are referred to my clinic are already on thyroid replacement medications for their hypothyroidism, however antibodies to the thyroid such as thyro-peroxidase antibodies (TPO) and thyroglobulin antibodies (TGLB), were never checked, so patients do not know they have an autoimmune disease. Instead, they feel fatigued despite having adequate thyroid hormone replacement and they don't know why this is happening. If you have a thyroid condition, I recommend you request checking TPO and TGLB antibodies if they haven't been done. If you have hyperthyroidism, a condition where too much thyroid hormone is produced, I recommend checking thyroid-stimulating immunoglobulin (TSI) antibodies as well.

Summary

- There is a strong gut-immune axis through the GALT, the gut-associated lymphoid tissue. Gastrointestinal symptoms are common people who have autoimmune disease, and in CFS patients.
- If you have an autoimmune syndrome and gastrointestinal issues, you will benefit from modifying the anti-inflammatory diet to include lectin-elimination. The most common lectins include gluten, soy, and kidney beans, which should be eliminated. Other lectins fall under the nightshade and legume family. Pressure cooking beans is a good way to eliminate lectins.
- Addressing IBS or dysbiosis can be helpful in calming down immune inflammation through the gut-immune axis and the gut-brain axis. Diagnostics include breath testing and microbiome testing.
- Some gastrointestinal doctors treat IBS and offer specialized testing. Most integrative or functional medicine doctors treat IBS and order specialized testing.
- Hashimoto's is the most common cause of hypothyroidism. Hashimoto's is an autoimmune condition diagnosed by the presence of antibodies against the thyroid. If you have hypothyroidism and have not had your antibodies checked, ask your doctor to check TPO and TGLB antibodies to confirm your status. If you have hyperthyroidism, have TSI antibodies checked too.
- COVID can cause an autoimmune condition to flare by raising general inflammation in the body even if this condition was well controlled in the past. COVID can even cause new autoimmunity to develop.
- An activated immune system is an inflamed immune system, and it contributes to fatigue symptoms.
- You can find a functional medicine practitioner in the Society of Functional Medicine (ifm.org/find-a-practitioner).

CHAPTER 7

Supplement Protocol for Long Haul

"Nutritional supplements are not a substitute
for a nutritionally balanced diet."
Deepak Chopra

N ow that you have a good understanding of the anti-inflammatory diet and hopefully an idea of what types of inflammation
you may have, you are ready to start the supplement protocol
for COVID Long Haul. Supplements can augment a healthy diet but are
not a substitute for it, and they cannot correct an unhealthy diet. Since
there is no known single therapy for COVID Long Haul, a holistic, natural approach may be most suitable for those still struggling with their
recovery. I have included the protocol below from Yanuck et al., which
includes 5 targets of support for COVID recovery. This protocol informed
my early practice with Long-COVID patients. As evidence for mast cell
activation emerged, I have modified it to include greater antihistamine
support. We will focus on the first two targets: foundational anti-inflammatory and antioxidant support, then add mast cell activation support
with bromelain, quercetin, and perilla.

In Figure 18, dosing is explained by QD, BID, TID, or QID. These are
commonly used to explain frequency. QD is Latin for "*quaque die*" or
once daily, BID means bi-daily or twice daily. TID means thrice daily,
and QID means quarterly daily, or four times daily. I have simplified
the recommendations with friendly bullet points at the end of this
chapter. I will go over each nutrient in the protocol to explain its
importance.

Figure 19. FIVE TARGETS OF SUPPORT FOR COVID

	PREVENTION	INFECTION	ESCALATING INFLAMMATION	RECOVERY
Foundation	Address Sleep, Stress, Diet (sugar, alcohol) Vit D 0.5-10,000 IU; Vit A 5-10,000 IU; Zinc 60 mg; Vit C 1 gm in divided doses: Melatonin 3-10 mg; Quercetin 500 mg TID; Fish Oil 3 grams per day; High Potassium diet		Vit C to bowel tolerance or IVC; Add K+ 200 mg QID	
Antioxidant Support	N-Acetyl Cysteine Glutathione (GSH)	NAC 900 mg BID — NAC 900 mg TID	NAC 900 mg QID; GSH 500 mg QID / Consider Other Modes of Delivery	
	For supply concerns, consider saving GSH for rampant inflam. phase			
NK Cells Support	Choose any 2: Astragalus 500 mg BID/TID; Andrographis 400 mg BID/TID; Reishi 400 mg BID/TID	Emphasis During Infection	In those with ramping inflammation, emphasis shifts from supporting immune surveillance to reducing inflammation.	
	In those at greater risk, immune surveillance support may need to start at baseline			
Support Th1	Berberine 500 mg BID/TID; Baicalin 300 mg BID/TID; *Alternate Options*: Echinacea 500 mg BID/TID; Goldenseal 500 mg BID/TID	Emphasis During Infection		
Anti-inflammatory Support	Curcumin; Bromelain; *Alternate Options*: Resveratrol 2-400 mg BID/TID; Sulforaphane 200 mg BID/TID; Boswellia 400 mg BID/TID	Curcumin 500 mg TID/QID	Curcumin 1 g QID / Consider higher doses as needed; Bromelain 600-2,400 GDU between meals	

Used with permission: Yanuck, Pizzorno, et al. (2020).

Zinc

One of the most important minerals for the body is zinc. The zinc finger proteins are one of the most abundant groups of proteins and have a wide range of molecular functions. Zinc is important in supporting the immune system, glucose metabolism, the production of dopamine in the brain and therefore optimal support of brain function and mood. Zinc supports production of thymulin, a compound needed for good immune function. The thymus is a gland that functions like an academy for your immune system. It trains competent immune cells to recognize enemy from self. Therefore, the thymus gland protects you from developing autoimmunity. When T cells graduate, they leave the thymus academy and are ready to jump into action to defend you. Zinc is used up quickly by the immune system in the setting of both infection and inflammation, so most people I see in my clinic are zinc deficient. Dietary sources of zinc include clams, oysters and in lower amounts in crustaceans like shrimp. Unless you eat oysters at last 1-2 times weekly, you are likely not getting enough dietary zinc. Our fruits and vegetables are lower in zinc content in the modern age because of modern irrigation techniques and soil depletion. I once went to visit Sicily and I couldn't believe how tasty their tomatoes were. I did not feel the need to add salt or pepper, their tomatoes were so rich in flavor. Sicily has an active volcano, Mount Etna, that infuses the soil with rich mineral content which flows into the fruits and vegetables grown there. My guess is that the folks who live in Sicily are not deficient in many minerals. In fact, Sardinia, near the region, is one of the Blue Zones of the world.

Zinc is low or borderline in about 98% of the patients I see in my clinic. For most people, I recommend 30 mg of zinc picolinate, preferably on an empty stomach, to improve absorption. For Long COVID, I double that amount to 30 mg twice daily. I have found increased complaints of nausea and gastritis at the 50 mg dose or higher. However, 30 mg twice daily is well tolerated. I recommend aiming for a goal level of zinc around 100 mg/mL, and balancing zinc with the copper level so they are close to a 1/1 ratio.

Vitamin C

Along with zinc, vitamin C is another vitamin that is heavily used by the body during episodes of inflammation and when it is fighting infection. Vitamin C is an important antioxidant, and it supports white blood cell function. One of our main bacterial infection fighters are neutrophils, and neutrophils use an "oxidative burst" mechanism to fight microbes. It is much like how hydrogen peroxide can disinfect surfaces. White blood cells need vitamin C for their oxidative burst, thus people who have low vitamin C therefore have cellular immune dysfunction. Vitamin C can be obtained from citrus fruits like orange and lemon, as well as strawberries and Kiwi fruit. Because it is water soluble, vitamin C is used up quickly by the body and then excreted through the urine. For this reason, I recommend 1000 mg daily in two divided doses. There are liposomal forms that are long acting, at higher price point, for convenience. Vitamin C, together with quercetin, act as mast cell stabilizers. I discuss quercetin below.

Vitamin D

Unless you are taking vitamin D3, you are likely vitamin D deficient. Vitamin D is the sunlight vitamin and obtained by direct sun exposure. Our ancestors labored under the sun and had plenty of sun exposure. However, most of us work indoors, and have been confined during the pandemic. It should come as no surprise then that over 90% of people I check are vitamin D deficient unless they are on some form of vitamin D supplementation. Vitamin D is important for regulating inflammation, but also to support the brain and a "sunny" mood. Low vitamin D levels have been associated with increased inflammation, lower mood, and decreased resistance to infection. Studies show that low vitamin D levels were associated with increased COVID severity and death.[52]

The optimal amount of vitamin D can be obtained naturally by getting daily full body exposure to sunlight—this means arms, legs, and trunk. The time needed varies, but one rule mentions that you need exposure for 1/3 of the time it would take to get a sunburn every day. With this calculation, if you would get sunburnt after one hour of unprotected sun exposure, your daily sun exposure needed to get optimal vitamin D levels would be 20 minutes. If you live in sunny Hawaii and are a beach bum, this may be easy for you. But for the rest of us who are not so lucky to live in sunny paradise, it may be necessary to take vitamin D. Vitamin D is present in low levels in salmon and mushrooms but is mostly absent in food. Optimal levels should be in the upper limits of normal. Though different labs have different value ranges, in many academic centers, the value is 50 ng/ml. LabCorp and Quest labs have a different normal range, with an upper limit of normal of 100 ng/ml, so a value of 50 would indicate need for vitamin D supplementation. People over the age of 50, those who are overweight, and those with more skin pigmentation are less likely to make adequate amounts of Vitamin D from sunlight exposure. The pigment melanin protects the skin against sunburns by blocking the uptake of UV light, yet this protection decreases vitamin D production in the skin, too. I recommend vitamin D3 5000 units daily and checking your level after 3 months.

Vitamin A

Vitamin A deficiency is not as common as vitamin D deficiency, although it is an important nutrient in supporting immunity. Vitamin A is also known as retinoic acid because it was discovered in the human retina and it is an important nutrient for eye health. Retinoic acid is created by conversion of beta carotene, a vitamin found in foods like carrots and pumpkins, and it is converted by two enzymes coded by the gene BCMO1. Some may have lower amounts of these enzymes, in which case there is a need for intake of retinoic acid from organ meats such as liver, kidneys, cod liver oil, or a vitamin A supplement. Vitamin A levels can be measured by a simple blood test, and if you have had low vitamin A level, you would do well to include this important nutrient in your daily supplementation. It is important to monitor levels, as vitamin A toxicity can cause elevation of liver enzymes and visual changes. For those with Long-Haul symptoms and vitamin A deficiency, I recommend 10,000 units of daily vitamin A and follow up testing in 1 month.[53]

Quercetin

Quercetin is a bioflavonoid found in certain foods, like raw onions and capers, as well as many fruits and vegetables. Quercetin is a bioflavonoid that plants use to protect themselves against infection, so it has anti-microbial properties. Its anti-inflammatory properties include mast cell stabilization, and therefore has benefits in reducing side effects of histamine inflammation, along with the classical pathways of inflammation. A study comparing conventional drug therapies for mast cell stabilization like leukotriene inhibitors and Cromolyn found quercetin has superior mast cell inhibition as compared to drug therapy.[54]

Drug therapy can be very effective at reducing symptoms of mast cell activation; however, it is possible to develop tolerance. The therapy becomes less effective with time. Quercetin has immune modulation properties that do not reduce over time but have additive benefits the longer you are on it. Quercetin also has direct anti-viral properties against COVID-19 and has been clinically studied in COVID infection. Quercetin, therefore, is one of the key bioflavonoids in both the treatment of COVID and resolution of COVID Long Haul. Many of the symptoms of acid reflux, dizziness and postural tachycardia, nausea and flushing described in Long Haul can be associated with mast cell activation and histamine excess. Histamine belongs to an inflammatory pathway that is associated with interleukin 4 and interleukin 13, both of which have been elevated in COVID Long Haul, and in chronic fatigue syndrome/Myalgic encephalitis.[55] These cytokines activate the 3 types of white blood cells that release histamine granules into the bloodstream: Mast cells, basophils, and eosinophils. Interestingly, old books on home remedies for recovering from a pneumonia recommended that folks rub raw chopped onions on their chest to improve wheezing. Though it sounds painful, it is possible that breathing improved because of the skin's absorption of quercetin through the capillaries. It is far easier to ingest the active compound orally. Notably, quercetin is not very well absorbed because it is a fat-soluble flavonoid, so it must be taken with food or with a teaspoon of a healthy fat like olive or perilla oil. Quercetin dosing is 1500 mg daily in divided doses with food or fat. Liposomal quercetin is more effective and can be taken on an empty stomach. Since quercetin is a key flavonoid in this protocol, if you find a blend that contains quercetin, be sure you are getting full 1500 mg daily, no less.

Omega-3 Fats

Omega-3 is an essential fatty acid that is important for cellular function and metabolism. It also is an important anti-inflammatory that can decrease nuclear factor kappa beta (NFKB) a molecule that generates multiple pathways of inflammation involving many cytokines including interleukin 6. You could even say NFKB activation is the primary root of most inflammatory pathways in the body. Interleukin 6 activity can be indirectly traced by a high sensitivity CRP (c-reactive panel). Eicosapentaenoic acid (EPA) and docosahexaenoic acid (DHA) are the most bio-available of all omega-3's. EPA is important for mood, neurotransmitter support, and is cardioprotective. DHA is neuroprotective, supports memory, and decreases brain inflammation. Both decrease neuro-inflammation. Vegetable sources of omegas provide alpha-linolenic acid (ALA), and are found in flaxseeds, avocados, sunflower seeds, and walnuts. All are anti-inflammatory, but our body only converts between 1-5% of ALA to EPA and DHA, therefore plant-based omega 3's and sources of EPA/DHA are both needed. Therefore, I recommend 3 grams of EPA and DHA supplementation in addition to the anti-inflammatory diet. If you are vegan, there are vegan omegas made from sea algae that can be used for DHA. For those with signs of neuro-inflammation, I recommend the triglyceride form of DHA or the phospholipid form of DHA, as it is more bioavailable in the brain. The free form of DHA, often present in the cheaper fish oils, enters the brain via passive diffusion mechanism. In brains that have an impaired blood brain barrier, this passive diffusion mechanism is also impaired, meaning less DHA will reach the brain where it can calm inflammation. The phospholipid form of omegas uses a different channel of entry making it a superior form for those suffering from neuroinflammation. For COVID, I recommend 3 grams daily. For daily health prevention, 2 grams are sufficient.

Turmeric

Another anti-inflammatory that blocks the inflammatory NFKB pathway is turmeric. The active compound in this yellow spice is called curcumin. Turmeric has been well studied in the scientific literature for its anti-cancer and anti-inflammatory properties. Turmeric is poorly absorbed into the body by the digestive tract; however, a small dash of pepper increases its bioavailability by 80%. For this reason, most turmeric supplements already add black pepper or a pepper extract, known as bioperine. If you choose to cook with turmeric, remember to add a dash of pepper to increase the bioavailability. Adding a fat, such as when you add coconut milk to a curry, also improves the bioavailability. I recommend 1-2 grams daily in divided doses. In larger doses turmeric can cause either constipation or diarrhea, so if this happens, reduce the dose to 1 gram daily or less.

Resveratrol

Resveratrol is another potent anti-inflammatory. There is excellent scientific data on the benefits of resveratrol in its role as an anti-inflammatory. It blocks NFKB but also activates sirtuin pathways in the body that have been linked to anti-aging benefits.[56] For those who cannot tolerate turmeric, resveratrol is a good alternative option. Resveratrol has some unique challenges to keep in mind, otherwise it will not have an impact at all. The first thing to remember is that resveratrol requires fat to be absorbed by the body. If you drink a resveratrol supplement with a cup of water, it will not be absorbed at all, and you will feel no benefit from your efforts. It is also important to obtain the *trans*-resveratrol form. Most of the supplements available commercially are simply titled resveratrol, which is in the *cis*-resveratrol form. That form of resveratrol is also not bioavailable to the body, even if taken with a dose of fat. Research on resveratrol has studied a wide variety of dosing. As with drugs, dosing is important for natural supplements. Most commercially available *trans*-resveratrol supplements are dosed at 150-200mg which is a small dose and possibly ineffective. Research conducted at Harvard supports 1 gram daily for adults.[57] The Long-Haul protocol recommends 400 mg 2-3 x daily, which is equivalent to 800-1200 mg daily. I opt for a resveratrol powder I can mix with a fat such as coconut yogurt or a high-quality olive oil, or a sublingual tablet that dissolves under the tongue. Suggested dosing of *trans*-resveratrol is 400 mg 2-3 x daily, with food or fat.[58]

Melatonin

Melatonin is much more than a sleep hormone. Your pineal gland produces between 0.5-0.8 mg of melatonin at night, as a signal that it is time to go to bed. As we get older, production of many hormones, including melatonin, decreases. Melatonin has immune regulating effects and anti-inflammatory effects on the brain in addition to its benefits for sleep initiation. For insomnia, I normally recommend physiologic doses, between 0.5-1 mg at bedtime. My pet peeve is that most over-the-counter brands do not have the correct physiologic dosing, instead selling 5 and 10 mg doses. People try the larger doses and wake up feeling hungover the next day. This dose is too high! For people not used to taking melatonin, I recommend starting with 1 mg at bedtime, then increasing to 3 mg after 1 week, if tolerated, eventually increasing to 5 mg. Melatonin can decrease brain inflammation, so higher doses are used for Long COVID. If an increased dose causes drowsiness the next morning, lower the dose by ½.

Potassium

The western diet is a diet high in salt and sugar and low in zinc, potassium, and magnesium. However, too much sodium is pro-inflammatory. A high potassium diet is anti-inflammatory, as cells require potassium clear intra-cellular debris and toxins. Sodium is exchanged for potassium and other essential minerals like calcium in the renal tubules of the kidneys. As explained in the anti-inflammatory diet, it is important to balance sodium with also potassium content in the diet. One easy way is to exchange your saltshaker for a salt alternative and cook with a potassium chloride salt. There is a 50/50 salt alternative that combines sodium and potassium in equal measures. Patients with chronic kidney disease or on dialysis should not take potassium supplements unless recommended by their kidney specialist.

NAC (N-Acetylcysteine) Versus Glutathione

Remember the right and left hand of lowering inflammation, which must include antioxidants? When oxidative stress from free radicals overwhelms our liver's ability to neutralize and eliminate them, these toxins bind to cells and damage them, creating more oxidative stress and damage. This can be a source of ongoing inflammatory drive that doesn't resolve. The liver detoxifies our bodies by producing superoxide dismutase, a free radical neutralizer, and glutathione, a toxin binder, as two of our main detoxification pathways. N-acetylcysteine (NAC) is the precursor of glutathione, and the cofactor needed to produce glutathione is zinc and selenium. Brazil nuts are the highest dietary source of selenium. NAC additionally has evidence that it breaks down biofilms, allowing the immune system to find and eliminate more viruses hiding behind biofilm membranes. If you choose to take glutathione, remember that it is not very bioavailable, so for improved absorption, take glutathione with food or fat, or purchase the liposomal form. NAC is water soluble, so it's an easier form to take. There are some people who have lower levels of the enzyme needed to convert NAC to glutathione, and they will feel more benefits from taking liposomal glutathione. The COVID Long-Haul protocol includes high doses of NAC, of up to 2.7 grams daily in divided doses along with adequate dietary selenium, in the form of 2 Brazil nuts daily. I you prefer to use liposomal glutathione; the recommended dose is up to 2 grams daily in divided doses. You can start with lower doses and gradually increase as tolerated.

Case 2: "Paul" (name changed) is a 38-year-old previously healthy computer engineer who worked at a startup in San Francisco. He developed COVID in the summer of 2021 and developed severe fatigue, brain fog, insomnia, shortness of breath, palpitations, and dizziness upon standing. He also developed increased anxiety and an impending sense of doom. We started the anti-inflammatory diet and supplements to lower inflammation, and he felt somewhat better initially, but after 3 months, his improvement reached a plateau. He remained fatigued enough that he had to take a leave of absence from work. On follow up, I saw he was not taking the full dose of NAC or quercetin as prescribed, so we discussed full dosing. Even though his serum histamine and tryptase levels were normal, I suspected mast cell activation. He responded to a trial of Pepcid, a histamine blocker, but the benefits faded after a couple of weeks. In the next follow-up visit, we added the mast cell protocol, adding full dose quercetin, bromelain, vitamin C and adding perilla. This modification turned his symptoms around. He felt well enough that he visited family in New York and was helping his father with gardening when he unfortunately developed COVID yet again. Since he was already on the protocol, he recovered rather quickly the second time around. His sense of doom was relieved by the breathwork and long walks in the forest. He remains on the mast cell protocol to this day.

TIPS for Supplements

Remember the fat-soluble supplements: glutathione, quercetin, and resveratrol? They need to be taken with food or fat or purchased in liposomal form, which includes fat in the capsule. Taking the supplements with water on an empty stomach is likely to result in zero benefits because they won't be absorbed.

Ensure you are buying a supplement labeled "GMP." This stands for good manufacturing practice, a stamp of quality. Supplements from Europe, where there is better regulation of industry, can serve as a trusted source and are increasingly available on online platforms such as Amazon and Vitacost.

Dosing is as important for supplements as it is for drugs. Taking too low doses due to pill burden or a desire to cut costs will cause disappointing results, or no effect at all. Do not skimp out on quercetin, as it is key for antihistamine support. Because natural supplements are not as bioavailable as pharmaceutical drugs, there are some inefficiencies, and taking low doses may result in minimal to no absorption. If you have a history of sensitivity to supplements, you may start with a low dose and go up slowly. Stop at the dose you can tolerate if the full dose is not tolerated.

Pregnancy

Botanicals as a group have not been studied in pregnancy and should be avoided. Vitamins like vitamin D, B2 and iron are safe and are recommended if you have low levels. Have your primary care doctor monitor your vitamin levels periodically if you are supplementing, to prevent over-correction.

Anticoagulants

If you are on anticoagulation therapy like Coumadin, Plavix or Eliquis, for a blood clot or heart condition, avoid this protocol. Botanicals and anti-inflammatory supplements as a group have properties which inhibit platelet aggregation, much like aspirin does. This is normally a good thing, but if you are on anticoagulants, there is an increased risk of bruising and bleeding. Consultation with an integrative medicine physician is advised to modify the protocol.

Liver Problems

If you have active hepatitis or liver failure, avoid this protocol, unless approved by your doctor. Some supplements are metabolized by the liver and the protocol may need to be adjusted to prevent more stress on your liver.

Histamine

If you suspect you have histamine intolerance, Th2 dominance or mast cell activation, add Perilla 150 mg twice daily to the protocol with the quercetin/bromelain/vitamin C combination (QBC). A preparation with liposomal quercetin will be superior since you can take liposomal quercetin on an empty stomach.

There are several commercially available combination supplements that include quercetin/bromelain/zinc and vitamin C to reduce pill burden. One is Solaray's QBC plex, and Orgabay's Liposomal Quercetin is another. Both are commercially available on Amazon.

There are few quality or reputable supplements for Perilla. The only two that I have found to be effective are: Pure Encapsulations Perilla and Metagenics Perimine, despite their higher price point. I have no commercial kickbacks with any of these companies, and I have no financial incentives in making these recommendations.

Summary of the Long-COVID Protocol

Basic Protocol
- Quercetin 1500 mg daily in divided doses
- Vitamin C 1000 mg daily in divided doses
- Zinc picolinate 30 mg twice daily
- Melatonin 3-6 mg at night (the optimal dose is unknown)
- Vitamin D3 5000 u/day–increase as needed to achieve a high normal range.
- NAC 1500-2700 mg daily in 2-3 divided doses
- Turmeric 1000-2000 mg in divided doses. Alt: Resveratrol 1000 mg daily (with fat/food)
- Omega-3 (either fish oil or vegan algae oil 3 grams daily in divided doses
- Low salt (2.3 grams) and high potassium (except for kidney impairment) anti-inflammatory diet.
- Optional: Famotidine 40mg BID (reduce dose with kidney impairment)

Basic Protocol with Added Mast Cell Stabilization
- (Mast Cell Support = QBC + Perilla)
- Quercetin 1500 mg daily in divided doses (liposomal preferred)
- Bromelain 1200 units-2400 units in between meals
- Vitamin C 1000 mg in divided doses
- Perilla 150 mg twice daily (suggested Perilla brands: Pure Encapsulations or Metagenics)
- Zinc picolinate 30 mg twice daily
- Melatonin 3-6 mg at night (the optimal dose is unknown)
- Vitamin D3 5000 u/day–increase as needed to reach the upper normal levels.
- NAC 1500-2700 mg daily in 2-3 divided doses
- Omega-3 (either fish oil or vegan algae oil) 3 grams daily in divided doses
- Low salt (2.3 grams) and high potassium (except for renal impairment) anti-inflammatory diet
- Optional: Famotidine 40mg BID (reduce dose with renal impairment)

Optional for Mast Cell Activation
If you are intolerant to either quercetin of bromelain, choose 3 mast cell activators to combine with Perilla. For example, you can substitute bromelain with astragalus, rutin, or luteolin below. Since bromelain has anti-clotting

activities, consider adding another clot-buster such as nattokinase or serra-peptase. If levels of B2 and ferritin are low, correct those nutrients as well.

- Astragalus 1 gram twice daily
- Rutin 50 mg daily
- Luteolin 50 mg daily
- Vitamin B2 100-200 mg daily if low
- Vitamin B3 25-50 mg daily: start with 25 mg of niacin to prevent niacin flush. Alt: can use NAD+ or NMN.
- Iron Bis-glycinate 25 mg twice daily if ferritin below 100
- Consider adding Benadryl or Vistaril at bedtime to support sleep.

Tests to Consider

- Zinc/copper balance
- CRP
- ESR
- Ferritin
- B2
- B3 (if available)
- Vitamins A
- Vitamin D
- Plasma Histamine level (avoid antihistamines like Benadryl or acid blockers like Pepcid for 3 days before any blood test for histamine)
- Tryptase level

Weaning off the Protocol

The supplementation regimen described above can be challenging for some because of the number of pills that need to be taken daily. I usually warn patients they may need to take a modestly large number of supplements pills initially. Unfortunately, there is no "COVID multivitamin" that contains all the ingredients in the recommended doses and thus this regimen must be put together piecemeal, and there is some inefficiency. There are several Quercetin/bromelain/vitamin C/zinc combinations in the market, which can be helpful in reducing supplement burden. There is no combination that contains all the ingredients currently. Some people can experience supple-ment fatigue. Once people feel better, they feel the pill burden is worth it. However, once they feel back to their old self, patients invariably ask when they can stop the supplements.

A general rule of thumb is to expect a slower recovery if someone has had Long Haul for a year or more. It is almost as if the body had accepted inflam-mation to be the new normal and needs more convincing to turn things around. In this scenario, it may take several months on this protocol to feel back to baseline, but each month will see improvements in baseline energy and symptoms. It is also possible to have symptomatic flares during this time, but each will be milder and of a lesser duration. The overall trend will be one of progress. Patients who start this protocol four weeks after getting COVID can expect a much faster recovery and may feel better after just a couple of weeks. Each person's response will vary according to their co-existing medical conditions, and some people will need longer support than others. I recommend continuing the supplementation until you feel back to baseline, and then continuing for another 8 weeks. Remember that the recovery is being supported by use of the anti-inflammatory supplements. Stopping everything may cause rebound inflammation and backtracking in your recovery, much the same way some patients experience a rebound in inflammation after stopping a course of steroids.

After you feel back to baseline, wait 1-2 months before cutting the dosing of each supplement by ½. If your symptoms reappear after cutting the doses in ½, you are not ready to wean yet. Continue anti-inflammatory support for another 2 months. If after weaning there is no backsliding into your Long-COVID symptoms, you are ready to continue the weaning process. I recommend cutting doses by ½ every 2 months as tolerated until you no longer need to be on the protocol.

Summary

- The protocol for Long COVID addresses classic inflammation with anti-inflammatories such as vitamin D3 and fish oil.
- The protocol addresses oxidative stress by recommended antioxidants such as NAC or glutathione.
- The protocol for Long COVID addresses mast cell activation with quercetin, vitamin C, bromelain, perilla. Optional: add astragalus.
- Stay on the protocol until you return to baseline health, then continue for at least two more months. You can then taper doses of supplements slowly by ½ every 2 months. If you flare when tapering, you need to go back to the higher dose and stay there for another 2 months.
- Request testing for specific nutritional deficits and inflammatory markers. These include ferritin, vitamin D, B2, histamine, CRP, zinc, vitamin A, histamine, tryptase. Vitamin D levels should ideally be near the upper limits of normal.

CHAPTER 8

Nutrient Deficiencies

"You've gotta nourish to flourish."
Julie Stuckey

In the United States, we consume a calorie rich, nutrient poor diet. Foods are high is sugar, salt, and carbohydrates, yet often low in minerals like zinc, magnesium, potassium, and calcium, or needed nutrients like omega-3 fatty acids. People who follow a restricted diet because of underlying health conditions of who are vegan should know the gaps in nutrients and supplement accordingly. If you are vegan, I encourage you to become an informed vegan, so that nutrient deficiencies do not sneak up on you and cause cellular and metabolic dysfunction. Please see "7 Questions for Vegans" in Appendix 9, adapted from work published by Dr. Plotnikoff. I suspect that a subset of previously healthy people who developed Long Haul after COVID infection may not have resolved their inflammation due to deficiencies in certain nutrients. Studies have linked vitamin D deficiency to poorer outcomes in COVID infection, for example.[59] Infection and inflammation cause rapid consumption of several nutrients besides vitamin C and zinc. If these nutrients are not repleted, the body may run out of fuel for several metabolic healing processes.

We already discussed the lack of zinc and vitamin D and the need for supplementation in most diets in the chapter on the anti-inflammatory diet. Omega-3 ratios are often poor in a diet that lacks frequent fatty fish intake. There are a few other scenarios which increase the risk of developing nutrient deficits.

Vegan/Vegetarian Diet

If you are vegan, please become aware of the common nutrient gaps. Vegan diets are low in B12, B6, B7, B8, iron, essential amino acids including

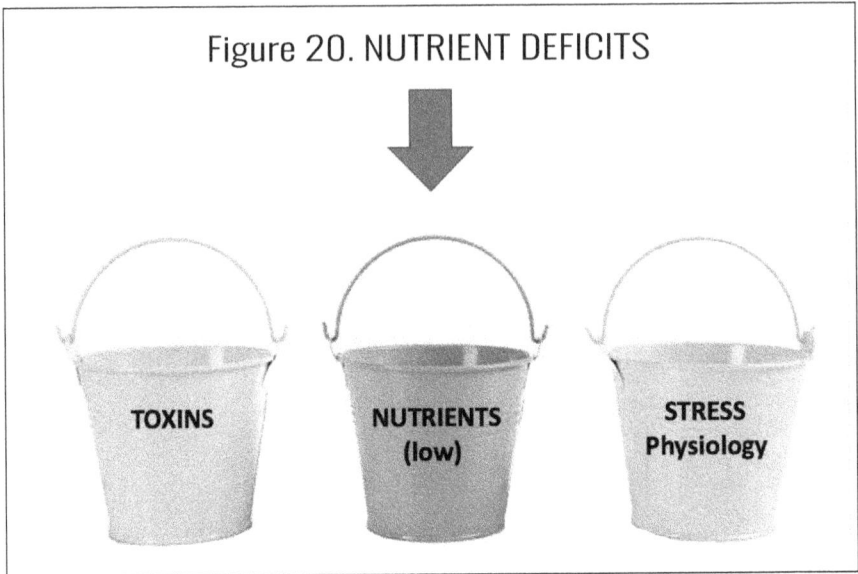

Figure 20. NUTRIENT DEFICITS

TOXINS

NUTRIENTS
(low)

STRESS
Physiology

tryptophan, leucine, isoleucine, valine, Vitamin D3 and omega-3 fatty acids, particularly EPA and DHA coming primarily from fish. Many fatigued vegans I encounter mistakenly believe that the omega-3 oils coming from flax and hemp seeds are sufficient, but this is false. Dietary conversion of the plant omega 3s known as ALA to the bioavailable EPA/DHA is low. This conversion takes place via a series of enzymatically controlled steps involving elongase and gamma-desaturase enzymes. Efficiency is estimated to be ≈5% for EPA and <0.5% for DHA. Not much! If you are vegetarian or vegan, consider supplementation with fish oils or algae-based omega-3 supplements which contain DHA and some EPA, besides incorporating plant sources of omega-3 fatty acids. EPA and DHA are not present in plant foods yet remain essential in lowering the inflammatory drive of NFKB.

Complete protein intake includes all the essential and conditionally essential amino acids. Essential amino acids are protein building blocks that our body cannot make, so we must consume them in the diet, and those at risk in a vegan or vegetarian diet include lysine, tryptophan, and methionine. There are few foods which are complete proteins besides animal meats. Examples include eggs, quinoa and freekeh. There aren't many in the plant realm.

Complete protein intake can come from eating a combination of beans, grains, nuts and seeds or tahini, as well as supplements such as Bragg's Amino Acids.

Diets rich in grains, corn, nuts, and seeds will be low in lysine. Lysine is found in legumes (beans, peas, and peanuts). Low appetite, weight loss, poor muscle tone, weakness and anemia can result from lysine deficiency.

Lysine is necessary for serotonin production and carnitine production (for beta-oxidation of fats and proteins). Notably, Lysine has anti-viral effects against infections with viruses from the herpesvirus family, including EBV and HSV, and which commonly reactivate in Long COVID, causing neuroinflammation. Lysine supplementation can be helpful in reducing viral load and viral reactivation of these viruses. (Please see the viral reactivation chapter for more information.)

According to Dr. Gregory Plotnikoff, author of "7 Questions for Vegans," diets rich in soybeans and other legumes can be low in tryptophan, cysteine, and methionine. These amino acids can be found in eggs, grains, and seeds. For these reasons, a combination of foods is needed. Supplementation may be required. Tryptophan is the building block for both serotonin and melatonin and therefore needed for mood, energy, and sleep.

Methionine is necessary to produce multiple neurotransmitters (epinephrine, normetanephrine, melatonin) as well for metabolism of multiple nutrients, production of insulin, coenzyme A, glutathione, EPA/DHA, iodine, and calcium.

Low iron can be best studied by a ferritin assay. Low ferritin or borderline ferritin is relatively common in many fertile women, but more so in the vegetarian or vegan population. I recommend that the ferritin level be near 100 ng/mL, which is the middle range of normal, for optimal health. Low ferritin, which I consider being anything below 30 ng/mL, is often associated with cold hands, icy feet, exercise intolerance, chronic fatigue, muscle aches with minimal exertion, all symptoms attributed to fibromyalgia. We already discussed how important iron is for the enzyme that breaks down histamine, ALDH, in the histamine chapter.

When I encounter a vegetarian or vegan patient with fatigue or chronic pain, I order a nutritional panel to detect any nutrient gaps.

Recommended Initial Testing for Vegans/Vegetarians with Fatigue

- Fasting B12, Methylmalonic acid
- Vitamin D
- High sensitivity CRP (elevated in either vitamin D deficiency or if there is a lack of omega-3s)
- ESR
- Homocysteine
- Zinc/copper
- Ferritin
- Plasma amino acids
- Plasma histamine and tryptase

Women

Women are at higher risk for nutrient deficits. I diagnose many more vitamin deficiencies in women than in men. This may be partly because women have a lower caloric intake. The standard caloric intake for women is 1200-1500 Kcal and for men, the caloric intake averages 2000-2400 Kcal, nearly double. With twice the amount of food, men have a two-fold chance of meeting nutritional needs by sheer volume of intake. Hormonal therapies like birth control pills increase the risk of vitamin deficiencies in women. Hormonal therapies are metabolized by the liver and compete with metabolism of several B vitamins including B2, B12 and B6.[60] Last, women of a fertile age lose iron every month, and iron deficiency contributes to fatigue and histamine intolerance as we have already discussed.[61]

Medications

Some commonly prescribed medications can cause select nutritional deficiencies. Antacids in the proton pump inhibitor family, like omeprazole, pantoprazole, carry a black box warning that they should not be used for over four weeks. People often take them for much longer, even years. Gastric acid is needed for the absorption of many vitamins and, including calcium, magnesium, iron, and all the B vitamins. Statins, a family of drugs which are commonly prescribed to lower cholesterol, deplete the body of Coq10, a cofactor needed for delivery of electrons to the mitochondria, where it creates ATP—the energy currency of the body. In fact, the most common side effect of statins is severe muscle aching. This side effect is called myalgia; it results from depletion of bodily Coq10, and it can be corrected by prescribing Coq10 supplementation. When I see a patient on a statin drug, I recommend supplementing with Coq10 400 mg daily with food/fat in the first month, then 200 mg thereafter.[62]

Minerals

Our ancestors drank water from river streams. This water was rich in essential minerals such as calcium zinc, boron, and magnesium. Today, our chlorinated water is deficient in minerals. The same depleted water supplies irrigation of farms, making our vegetables lower in mineral content. Modern farming practices overuse the topsoil layer resulting in a nutrient poor plant. Consider adding trace minerals to your water regularly. You will feel more hydrated. Ideally, choose a trace minerals solution that doesn't have added sugar. Lastly, while I mentioned that iodine deficiency is rare in the United States, vegetarian diets are at higher risk for iodine deficiency especially if iodized salt is avoided in meal preparation.

Gastrointestinal Disorders

Poor absorption of nutrients can occur in people who have gastrointestinal disease. This is called malabsorption. Gastrointestinal inflammation can cause malabsorption of nutrients. Conditions such as bariatric surgery, colectomy or other bowel surgery, a history of colitis, celiac disease, bacterial overgrowth, inflammatory bowel disease or inflammatory bowel syndrome (IBS), are all at high risk. IBS is common, even in the absence of prior intestinal surgery. Studies estimate it affects up to 11%-25% of the population worldwide.[63] If you have a history of chronic diarrhea, consider a comprehensive gastrointestinal evaluation to see if you have developed impaired nutrient absorption

Low Stomach Acid

In some people, secretion of gastric acid decreases and may cause a condition called hypochlorhydria. This can contribute to poor vitamin absorption and indigestion. Paradoxically, low stomach acid can *cause* symptoms of reflux because the food sits in the stomach undigested. If food can't go down, it will come up. Many will then get prescribed antacids, which only make this condition worse. The correct solution is to take a digestive enzyme containing betaine HCL with food. You can try a simple home test called the "baking soda test" to see if this applies to you. First thing in the morning in a fasting state, mix ¼ teaspoon of baking soda into a cup of water. Drink on an empty stomach. If you have stomach acid, the baking soda will react with your gastric acid to produce carbonation, resulting in burping within a few minutes. Much in the same way a carbonated drink would affect you. This is a normal test. If you don't burp, you may lack stomach acid and would benefit from a digestive enzyme containing betaine HCL. Causes of low gastric acid can include H. Pylori infection, antibodies against parietal cells, and age over 50. You can have these antibodies checked by your primary care physician if your home acid test is abnormal.[64]

You can see how a woman who is vegan, takes prescription antacids and/or hormonal therapies, or has signs of IBS would be at high risk for developing fatigue from several nutrient deficits.

Dories story: Dorie (name altered) is a delightful 70-year-old woman referred to me for chronic fatigue lasting 20 years. Dorie was remarkably healthy for her age, ate a healthy Mediterranean diet, and took only one medication for her blood pressure at a low dose. She was previously an avid hiker, loved biking and being active in her community by volunteering. Dorie initially associated her fatigue with getting older, but as it progressed over the decades, she found she could no longer get out of bed. I checked a baseline nutrient panel and found she was severely deficient in vitamin D3,

B 12, and her ferritin was rock bottom. She did not have anemia, but her ferritin level was 13ng/mL (12 was the cut-off). I started her on a regimen of iron bis-glycinate, vitamin D, and B 12. Dorie experienced a dramatic improvement in her fatigue after just two weeks of correcting her nutrient deficiencies and started enjoying her outdoor activities again.

In Dorie's case, I suspect her iron had been low for the past 20 years, when the fatigue started. No one had checked it in two decades. Because of her fatigue, she was not out in the sun with her usual activities, and she became vitamin D deficient as well. Dorie is unique among my patients in that her fatigue came from a single bucket: nutrient deficits. Because we did not need to address other buckets, her improvement was quick and dramatic. It is a shame she had to wait so long to have someone check her vitamin stores!

Summary

- Vegan and strict vegetarian diets are at risk for several nutritional deficiencies, including amino acid deficiencies and deficiencies in iron, EPA/DHA. If you are vegan, please read the handout "7 questions for Vegans" in the appendix section. Consider a multivitamin containing iron and amino acid supplementation with either Bragg's Aminos, or amino acid capsules.
- Minerals are low in the western diet. Consider adding trace minerals to your water that include potassium, calcium, magnesium, and zinc besides sodium.
- Women are at higher risk of nutritional deficits due to numerous factors. They include lower caloric intake, as women generally consume ½ the calories that men do. Use of hormonal therapies such as birth control can increase risk of several B vitamin deficits. Women are at higher risk for iron deficiency as well.
- Gastrointestinal inflammatory conditions such as celiac disease, inflammatory bowel disease or inflammatory bowel syndrome can cause poor absorption of nutrients, resulting in vitamin deficits. Loose stools or frequent diarrhea should prompt clinical evaluation by your primary care doctor or a gastroenterologist.
- Medications such as long-term use of antacids like proton pump inhibitors (Omeprazole, Pantoprazole) and histamine blockers (Famotidine/Pepcid) increase the risk of vitamin deficiency since many vitamins need stomach acid for absorption. Medications for cholesterol like statins can cause select nutrient deficits of Coq10.

- Some people develop a condition called hypochlorhydria—low gastric acid levels resulting in impaired absorption of vitamins. A simple home bicarbonate test can test that theory (see the appendix section for the home bicarbonate test). Hypochlorhydria can paradoxically cause reflux symptoms, and it can be treated with supplementation of betaine hydrochloride. Antacids like Omeprazole or famotidine only make this condition worse and should be avoided.

CHAPTER 9

Neuroinflammation, Vagal Tone, and Stress Physiology

"Feelings come and go like clouds in a windy sky.
Conscious breathing is my anchor."
Zen Buddhist monk Thick Nhat Hahn

Neuroinflammation is common in Long COVID and can cause feelings of brain fog, headaches, shifts in mood, and increased stress physiology. During a cytokine storm such as the one that occurs with COVID, there is one central brain pathway that can be derailed, leading to promotion of central nervous system inflammation, and thus whole-body inflammation. This pathway is linked to the fight-or-flight system and is known as the autonomic nervous system (ANS).

The vagus nerve is susceptible to becoming weaker with exposure to inflammation, or because of an inflammatory cytokine surge such as that occurring in COVID.[65] It is not uncommon for people recovering from COVID to report that they have more trouble controlling a sense of dread, panic, and anxiety due to increased stress physiology. Simple things like getting through a phone call may leave them with palpitations and sweats. Therefore, to fully recover from Long COVID we must also address how to decrease stress physiology. This can be accomplished by engaging in neurorehabilitation of the vagus. I will refer to weak vagal tone as vagal dystonia from now on. Vagal toning can be considered "Pilates for your vagus" in much the same way you might need to strengthen your core muscles upon your recovery. Thus, vagal toning is a key component of full recovery from Long Haul.[66]

86

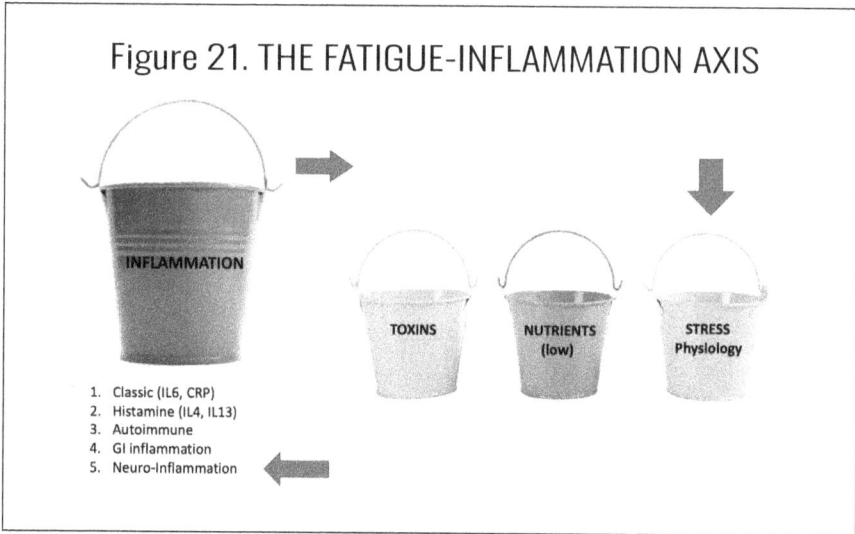

Figure 21. THE FATIGUE-INFLAMMATION AXIS

INFLAMMATION

TOXINS

NUTRIENTS (low)

STRESS Physiology

1. Classic (IL6, CRP)
2. Histamine (IL4, IL13)
3. Autoimmune
4. GI inflammation
5. Neuro-Inflammation

The vagus is an unusual and interesting nerve. It is the only nerve that ventures out of the safety of the protected skull and wanders through the front and center of the body. It is therefore appropriately named *Vago* in Latin meaning "wanderer." As the vagus wanders through the front of the body, it connects with various organs: the voice box, the heart, the lungs, the stomach, the diaphragm, the bowels, as well as the spleen and liver. It has major regulatory functions in each of these organs. Many of the symptoms that Long-COVID sufferers report are related to vagal dystonia, such as tachycardia, increased stomach acid and digestion troubles, difficulty breathing, and problems with blood pressure.

Vagal outflow tract fibers connecting to the lungs and diaphragm have stretch receptors. Therefore, stretching your lungs and diaphragm through deep, held breaths is an easy way to rehabilitate the vagus. I recommend the 4-7-8 breath to all my patients. Dr. Andrew Weil has an excellent video showing the technique—drweil.com/videos-features/videos/breathing-exercises-4-7-8-breath/.

The 4-7-8 breath should be carried out twice a day, and it only takes 1 minute of time. There is no reason to not do this breath even if you are busy. Think of the 4-7-8 breath technique as "Pilates for your vagus." Just two repetitions a day will make a big difference in a couple of months. Addressing the physiologic stress caused by vagal dystonia and runaway activation of the central nervous system is key to your recovery.

Another great resource is the free online COVID recovery group called Stasis—stasis.life. This group focuses on Long-COVID recovery by engaging breath work and mindfulness-based approaches to reduce stress. There are optional personal one-on-one sessions at cost, however, many of my patients listen to the free educational modules and videos. Mindfulness-based stress reduction (MBSR) has volumes of research in stress physiology and is also recommended, though most good courses cost a few hundred dollars.

The vagus acts much like a brake pad on the fight-or-flight system. You can imagine with vagal dystonia, how it could be difficult to control fight-or-flight and reign in stress physiology. This is analogous to an old car with old brake pads that keeps moving after you hit the brakes. It is harder to control. Vagal toning is akin to changing the brake pads for brand new ones. Now you can control the car and break whenever necessary.

Our central nervous system has been wired to go into fight or flight in a split second. From an evolutionary standpoint, this makes sense; survival takes precedence over everything else, even if it sacrifices health and longevity. The most important thing evolutionarily is to survive long enough to have offspring. If you think about our cave dweller ancestors, when facing a predator, an instant surge of epinephrine, cortisol, and adrenalin to outrun and outsmart the predator is highly advantageous. To achieve this, the ANS baseline mode is to be in fight-or-flight. Vagal tone acts as a brake pad on the fight or flight accelerator. The moment the vagal stop lifts, you are off to the races. But what if your vagal tone is weak? Now you have a runaway car that you cannot control. Since runaway stress physiology promotes inflammation, this becomes a loop of self-reinforcing inflammation. Stress physiology consumes important energetic resources, contributing to symptoms of fatigue.

The engagement of breath work and mindfulness to rehabilitate the vagus is therefore the final and key step needed in ensuring full recovery from Long COVID. There are, fortunately, many ways to strengthen the vagal tone.

Mindfulness meditation, guided imagery, and mindfulness-based stress reduction are helpful interventions with multiple clinical studies. Ear acupuncture can be helpful because of vagal outflow receptors present in the deeper concave portion of the ear, known as the conchae of the ear. Studies of veterans using "battlefield acupuncture" a type of acupuncture that includes embedded vagal studs in the ear, have shown long-term stress reduction. Apps like Headspace, CALM, and Insight timer have pre-loaded guided meditations. I encourage you to explore several avenues in besides the 4-7-8 breath, and to consider adopting a mindfulness practice of at least 10-minutes a day.

Spending time in nature, or forest bathing, can do wonders to calm the central nervous system. Forest bathing is called shinrin yoku in Japan and it is a common health-promoting practice. Studies on transcutaneous vagal stimulation in acute COVID and have been linked to drastically reduced inflammatory interleukin 6 levels.[67] Transcutaneous vagal stimulation is currently being studied in Long COVID in at least 6 current clinical studies.

Supplements like choline and huperzine support healthy vagal function.

Choline is a precursor of the neurotransmitter acetylcholine, and it has many important functions in the body, including being the main neurotransmitter of the vagus, so it's important in digestive health too.[68] Huperzine—from Huprezia Serrata, a fir moss plant extract—inhibits the breakdown of choline in the body, and it is another way to increase choline in the brain.[69] Choline has other important functions in the body, such as improving bile flow and supporting liver detoxification.[70] Choline has some anti-histaminic and anti-inflammatory properties as well. You can see why it is one of my favorite supplements.[71] Huperzine is dosed at 10 mg daily, and I like to recommend phosphatidylcholine dosed at 600 mg twice daily, preferably with meals, since choline improves digestion through increased bile flow. Genetics can play a role in choline deficiency: the PEMT and MTHFD-1 genes are involved in choline production and allele variants of this gene are common, resulting in lower production of choline in the body. Dietary sources of choline include eggs and chicken liver.[72]

Glial cells are white blood cells near neurons, and they can become activated in COVID infection and in CFS.[73] Inactivated glial cells are like meek, timid scientists that keep neurons nourished and in good health. However, when glial cells become activated, they undergo a Hulk-like transformation. These activated, Hulk-like glial cells promote chaotic inflammation and even damage nearby neurons in their fury. Low-dose naltrexone (LDN) has been used to address neuroinflammation with success in many who have developed CFS because of glial activation. LDN has anti-inflammatory and glial regulating properties, so these white blood cells can go back to becoming placid scientists again. LDN is often titrated up slowly, starting with a dose of 0.5 mg, increased by 0.5 mg weekly over nine weeks until the final dose of 4.5 mg is reached.[74] Some patients experience dramatic results on LDN, others have a partial or no response. I suspect those who do not respond to LDN have unaddressed mast cell activation instead. Histamine is a bioactive amine in the brain that promotes inflammation through the secondary interleukin 4 pathway we discussed earlier. If you have tried LDN but not experienced any benefits, I suggest you try the mast cell activation protocol discussed in the previous chapter. LDN cannot be used if you are taking opioid medications since it binds to opioid receptors.

As mentioned previously, there are 100 million neurons in our gastrointestinal tract. A disordered gut can cause neuroinflammation through a vast connection of neurons that hard-wire the brain and the gut together. If you are experiencing gastrointestinal or digestive disruption, please consider being evaluated and treated for them by a gastroenterologist and possibly an integrative practitioner for a comprehensive evaluation. Seeing how the brain can be negatively affected by so many avenues of inflammation, it is not surprising that brain fog is the most common symptom in CFS and in Long COVID.

Last, if you experienced trauma during your COVID infection, or have unresolved past traumatic experiences, it is good to seek a therapist who is trained in trauma recovery. There are techniques such as the emotional freedom technique (EFT) and eye movement desensitization (EMDR) that are highly efficacious in processing trauma, so it can move the experience from your present awareness into a processed file in your knowledge bank. A therapist trained in trauma therapy will have access to these techniques and more. Once trauma is processed, it becomes easier to lower physiologic stress, improve vagal tone, and conserve energy. A strong vagal tone has health promoting and anti-inflammatory effects on both brain and body.

Summary

- Neuroinflammation is common in Long COVID. Neuroinflammation can be caused by vagal dystonia, glial activation, and/or mast cell activation.
- Neuroinflammation increases stress physiology in the body. Stress physiology reinforces inflammation and wastes vital energetic resources, resulting in fatigue.
- The vagus controls not only our autonomic nervous system; it regulates multiple organs in the body, making vagal toning key to recovery CFS and Long COVID. Consider vagal toning "Pilates for your vagus."
- Vagal toning can be accomplished in many ways: breathwork is the easiest, and mindful practices are encouraged. Forest bathing is useful too. Transcutaneous vagal stimulation has been studied in COVID and observed to lower inflammation.
- Start by practicing the simple 4-7-8 breath technique at least twice daily. You can find free COVID recovery mindfulness classes on the stasis.life website. Spend time in nature.
- Supplements to support the vagus include choline and Huperzine. Huperzine 10 mg daily and phosphatidylcholine choline 600 mg twice daily can be useful, especially in people with choline deficiency.
- Glial activation can cause neuroinflammation. LDN has been helpful in reducing glial activation and can be useful in a subset of CFS and Long-COVID patients. LDN is usually started at a dose of 0.5 and titrated up slowly until the maximum dose of 4.5 mg has been reached.
- Mast cell activation can produce neuroinflammation, making the mast cell protocol useful in another subset of patients, especially those who do not respond to LDN.

- There is a significant gut-brain connection. Addressing gastrointestinal inflammation has many benefits in reducing neuro-inflammation.
- Addressing trauma through trauma-informed therapy should be considered if it is contributing to stress physiology and vagal dystonia.

CHAPTER 10

Postural Autonomic Tachycardia (POTS)

"Getting old isn't for the faint of heart."
Mae West

A subset of patients will develop symptoms of dizziness upon standing, tachycardia, and a drop in their blood pressure, along with a racing heart sensation. This is termed "orthostatic" and it can happen weeks to months after COVID recovery. POTS is diagnosed when your heart rate increases by 30 beats a minute or more, usually within 10 minutes of standing. This increase in heart rate can last for over 30 seconds and can be associated with other symptoms such as weakness, dizziness, and panic or a sense of a racing heartbeat, even fainting. POTS can be diagnosed formally by a tilt table test, which requires a referral to cardiology by your primary care doctor. Symptoms which can mimic POTS can include dehydration, acute blood loss, adrenal insufficiency, hypoglycemia, or vasovagal syncope. Salt tablets and using minerals with sodium and potassium can be helpful in reducing symptoms by increasing blood pressure. Beta blockers such as propranolol and magnesium can be helpful in reducing palpitations. A newer drug, Ivabradine/corlanor, selectively slows the sinus node pacemaker of the without worsening low blood pressure in COVID Long Haulers. Compression stockings in the legs can help keep blood from pooling in the legs, and even abdominal binders can be helpful if you have difficulty with prolonged standing. you have difficulty with prolonged standing. Others have found Spanx compression undergarments to be more comfortable than abdominal binders. Many medical centers will have a cardiac rehab program for those who have a POTS diagnosis.[75]

If you have POTS, smaller and more frequent meals are better tolerated to reduce redirection of blood flow to the stomach. Making sure you keep activity gentle and prevent your heart rate from going above 110 beats per minute can be helpful to prevent post exertional fatigue. In the next chapter, I focus on the Dallas CHOP protocol for POTS patients, but I also recommend this graduated exercise program to all COVID Long Haulers since over-exertion is a common problem that sets people back on their recovery, and pacing is key to recovery.

Natural Approaches to POTS

Hydrate with trace minerals, not just water. Minerals such as salt, potassium and magnesium help to improve your overall hydration status, more than water alone. Salt tablets can be extremely useful.

The heart loves magnesium since magnesium is necessary for smooth muscle contractions. Magnesium also lowers heart rate and improves muscle contractility, an added benefit for those experiencing palpitations. Consider using at least 500 mg-1000 mg of magnesium daily. Magnesium is safe and non-toxic, the only side effect of too much magnesium is loose stools. I recommend escalating your magnesium dose gradually and stop when you notice an increased frequency of stools. If you notice loose stools at 1000 milligrams of magnesium, for example, consider going down on the dose by 200 mg. Magnesium oxide and citrate are more likely to cause loose stools, therefore magnesium glycinate or threonine are preferable since they are better absorbed. Start with at least 500 mg of magnesium daily and slowly go up from there.

Deglycyrrhizinated (DGL) Licorice is helpful in POTS by supporting adrenal function and recirculation of minerals due to its aldosterone-like effects. It supports blood pressure because of cortisol-like effects and is helpful if you suffer from low blood pressure. Doses recommended include 100-400 mg daily, not to exceed 800 mg daily. Licorice in doses over 400 mg should not be taken continuously for over 2 weeks unless potassium levels are being monitored, and it should be avoided in those with hypertension. The WHO suggests that most healthy adults can safely eat up to 100 mg per day of glycyrrhizin acid, or about 2–2.5 ounces (60–70 grams) of licorice.[76] DGL licorice is recommended over regular licorice because of toxicity associated with excessive glycyrrhizin intake.

Because our heart rate is regulated by the vagus, the vagal toning techniques mentioned in the chapter on neuroinflammation can be very helpful and are highly recommended.

As we saw in the mast cell activation chapter, mast cell activation or excess histamine can cause POTS symptoms, and histamine acts as a vasodilator.[77] If you have POTS, add the mast cell protocol with quercetin/bromelain/vitamin C/Perilla mentioned in the histamine protocol.

If you haven't already done so, consider being formally evaluated for

POTS with a tilt-table test. In such patients, low dose beta blockers like propranolol have been helpful in reducing some of the tachycardia and palpitations, along with adding salt and minerals to their water. Even if you do not have POTS but have symptoms like it, the recommendations in this book will help guide your recovery. Your PCP can help to refer you to the appropriate cardiovascular specialist.

Gradually increasing exercise and pacing of activities will be important. The graduated exercise protocol called Dallas-CHOP protocol for exercise intolerance will be discussed in the next chapter.

Summary

- Symptoms of dizziness upon standing, racing heart and drop in blood pressure upon standing may suggest POTS. POTS can be due to low blood pressure upon standing. Other causes include vasovagal syncope and hypoglycemia.
- POTS is suggested when your heart rate increases by 30 beats a minute or more, usually within 10 minutes of standing. It is diagnosed formally with tilt-table testing, which normally involves a cardiology referral. Beta blockers such as propranolol can be prescribed for tachycardia. If you suspect you have POTS, consider formal evaluation.
- Small, frequent meals are helpful to prevent blood from pooling in the digestive tract.
- Compression stocking and abdominal binders can help support blood pressure when standing.
- Salt tablets are highly useful in POTS. Hydration with trace minerals, including sodium, magnesium, and potassium, is more effective than drinking water alone.
- Magnesium can be very effective in reducing palpitations associated with POTS. Magnesium glycinate or magnesium threonate starting at 500 mg daily can be useful and titrated up for effect. Magnesium is very safe; the limiting dose is the one that causes loose stools (exception: patients with renal failure).
- DGL licorice can support adrenal function in POTs and helps to increase blood pressure. It has aldosterone-like effects, which means it can help with salt balance. Doses recommended include 100-400mg daily, not to exceed two weeks of use if using 400 mg or more, as it can cause potassium imbalances. After two weeks, consider having your potassium levels checked by your primary care doctor.
- Mast cell activation can cause POTS symptoms, consider adding the mast cell protocol described in the previous chapters.[78]
- Graduated exercise is important and will be described in the next chapter.

CHAPTER 11

Exercise Intolerance

"Slow and steady wins the race."
The Tortoise and the Hare
Aesop (c620-c560 B.C.)

One of the hardest things about Long COVID is the inability to exercise, and the worsening fatigue after exercise, known as post-exertional malaise. This is also a hallmark of CFS. After months of feeling ill and fatigued, once people finally start feeling better, they may go out for a walk to enjoy a sunny day, then feel like their recovery has been set back by several months. The reason for this setback goes back to our model of inflammation, described at the beginning of the book. Normally, in an uninflamed body, exercise is a hormetic stimulus. Hormesis means a small amount of stress which is good for you. Exercise causes a small amount of self-limited inflammation. Inflammation rises, then falls, and in doing so sets off a cascade of regeneration and cellular repair that are beneficial for the body.

In Long Haul there is too much unresolved inflammation. Even a small amount of exercise can be the straw that breaks the camel's back, and it re-inflames the body to levels that it cannot resolve, creating cellular damage. You feel terrible and malaise flares up. The payback is severe. It is very important to be patient with yourself during this process and apply a method of graduated exercise that is slow and progressive. Most people adopt the mindset of "no pain, no gain" when exercising. For Long-COVID and CFS sufferers, this is a big mistake. Pushing past signs of fatigue will delay your recovery by promoting a cycle of inflammation that is hard to resolve.

Pacing of activities is key. If you exert yourself, give yourself time to recovery. Don't push through the fatigue. Incorporate several periods of recovery

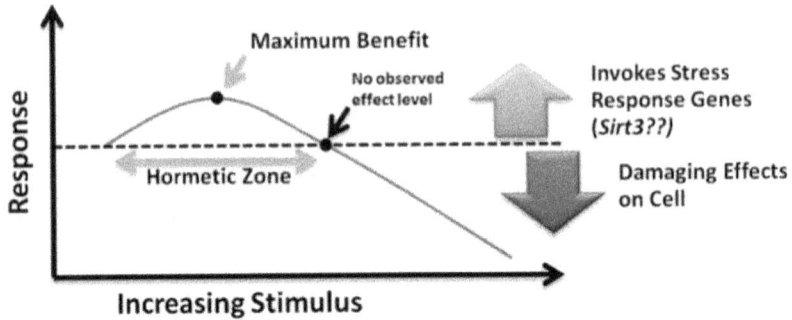

Figure 22. HORMETIC RESPONSE TO EXERCISE AND ROS

Adapted with permission: "Forever young: SIRT3: a shield against mitochondrial meltdown, aging, and neurodegeneration," researchgate.net/figure/hermetic-response-curve-within-the-hormetic-zone-mil-or-moderate-doses

within your daily activities. This is called "pacing." For example, if you are cleaning the house or cooking for 30 minutes, schedule 30 minutes for rest soon after. For exercise, I recommend the modified CHOP-POTS protocol of graduated activity. This protocol was developed at the University of Philadelphia for those diagnosed with POTS (Postural Tachycardia Syndrome). The protocol begins with floor exercises to build up core muscle strength in the abdomen and legs for the first month, followed by gentle, progressive aerobic exercise in a graduated, disciplined manner starting in a recumbent position. During this recovery period, you may think, "I'll never be able to exercise like I did before." I assure you with patience, and following this protocol, you will. Now is the time to be patient and start low, go slow. The new mindset you must adopt is "slow and steady wins the race." You will need to learn to listen to your body's signals of perceived exertion. You will need to unlearn the tendency to push yourself past the fatigue.[79]

In the CHOP-POTS exercise program, you can expect to exercise in the horizontal position for the first four months. Recumbent biking, rowing, or swimming laps are examples of recumbent exercises, and they alternate with days of strength training like Pilates exercises. In the fourth month, you can begin using an upright bike if available. On the fifth month, you may begin exercising upright with a treadmill, elliptical machine or even enjoy walking. It is recommended you keep watch over your heart rate with a heart rate monitor and watch over perceived exercise exertion. If you are on beta blockers for dysautonomia, you may need to rely on baseline heart rate and perceived exercise exertion more than your heart rate during exercise.

Figure 23 is an example of what month the first month might look like under the CHOP-POTS protocol.

Figure 23. MONTH 1 of CHOP-POTS PROTOCOL

Sunday	Monday	Tuesday	Wednesday	Thursday	Friday	Saturday
	Training Mode 1 5-10 min Warm Up / 3 min Base Pace / 2 min recovery / 3 min Base Pace / 5-10 min Cool down	Strength Training	**Training Mode 1** 5-10 min Warm Up / 3 min Base Pace / 2 min recovery / 3 min Base Pace / 5-10 min Cool down	Strength Training	**Training Mode 1** 5-10 min Warm Up / 3 min Base Pace / 2 min recovery / 3 min Base Pace / 5-10 min Cool down	
	Training Mode 1 5-10 min Warm Up / 4 min Base Pace / 3 min recovery / 4 min Base Pace / 5-10 min Cool Down	Strength Training	**Training Mode 1** 5-10 min Warm Up / 4 min Base Pace / 3 min recovery / 4 min Base Pace / 5-10 min Cool Down	Strength Training	**Training Mode 1** 5-10 min Warm Up / 4 min Base Pace / 3 min recovery / 4 min Base Pace / 5-10 min Cool Down	
	Training Mode 1 5-10 min Warm Up / 5 min Base Pace / 3 min recovery / 5 min Base Pace / 5-10 min Cool Down	Strength Training	**Training Mode 1** 5-10 min Warm Up / 5 min Base Pace / 3 min recovery / 5 min Base Pace / 5-10 min Cool Down	Strength Training	**Training Mode 1** 5-10 min Warm Up / 5 min Base Pace / 3 min recovery / 5 min Base Pace / 5-10 min Cool Down	
	Training Mode 1 5-10 min warm Up / 6 min Base Pace / 3 min recovery / 5 min Base Pace / 5-10 min Cool Down	Strength Training	**Training Mode 1** 5-10 min Warm Up / 7 min Base Pace / 3 min recovery / 5 min Base Pace / 5-10 min Cool Down	Strength Training	**Training Mode 1** 5-10 min Warm Up / 7 min Base Pace / 3 min recovery / 5 min Base Pace / 5-10 min Cool Down	

Training Mode 1 = any of supine cycling, recumbent bike, swimming laps with a kick board, rowing, seated stepper

Recovery = slow down, reduce resistance, get a drink, but don't stop moving.

Warm ups and cool downs are done starting very slowly with little or no resistance and leading up to and out of your Base Pace HR zone

Physical therapist can begin with supine cycling only if a patient is beginning program as wheel-chair bound/bedridden.

Weight training can be done on the same days as cardio workouts if necessary.

I have copied the step-by-step protocol directly from the University of Philadelphia website in the appendix section. All credit goes to the University of Philadelphia for making this protocol openly accessible to the public.

You can find more information about the CHOP Modified Exercise Program and download their step-by-step pdf here: dysautonomiainternational. org/pdf/CHOP_Modified_Dallas_POTS_Exercise_Program.pdf

If you decide to work with a physical therapist, ensure that you work with a therapist that is well versed in the CHOP-POTS protocol and has worked with POTS patients in the past. I have seen patient recovery derailed for months because a PT instructed them to work too hard, too fast, and push past the fatigue. The CHOP Modified Exercise Program is very cautious, and it is adequate for those who have just recovered from a COVID infection. If you can walk upright without any problems, you are past this initial recovery phase. In this case you are welcome to skip the first few months of the protocol start the upright exercise program.

Finally, please give yourself permission to be in this healing and recovery mode. Allow yourself to be in this growth stage—be patient and kind to yourself. There are important lessons you will learn that this phase will teach you. Move out any feelings of guilt and know that you will eventually emerge from this phase with a better understanding on how to heal your body.

Summary

- Exercise intolerance is common in both CFS and Long COVID.
- Pacing of activities and graduated exercise is key. Incorporate periods of rest after activity throughout the day and follow the CHOP-POTS protocol for graduated exercise.
- Consider following the mast cell activation protocol described in previous chapters.
- The new mindset is "slow and steady wins the race." Do not push through the fatigue but learn to listen to your body's signals and respect your current limitations.
- If you work with a physical therapist, be sure they are familiar with the CHOP-POTS protocol or POTS recovery to prevent setbacks.

CHAPTER 12

Adrenal Fatigue

"Trying to describe a good marriage is like trying to describe your
adrenal glands. You know they're in there functioning,
but you don't really understand how they work."
Helen Gurley Brown

Some Long-Haul symptoms of chronic fatigue may be from adrenal dysregulation, commonly referred to as "adrenal fatigue." It is possible for people to experience new insomnia with daytime fatigue, and a sensation of "doom." When energy is low in the body from high inflammation, the refined circuitry of the brain is impacted first, because it is one of the most active organs in the body and it requires high amounts of energy. An almond-sized gland in the brain called the hypothalamus regulates the adrenal glands down below, on top of the kidneys. The adrenals make chemicals that maintain daytime wakefulness such as cortisol and epinephrine. The adrenals also make aldosterone, a chemical that regulates salt balance, and they regulate sugar balance and sex hormone production. When the delicate interplay between the hypothalamus and the vagus is disrupted, it can cause a loss of circadian rhythm resulting in feelings identical to those of jetlag. Since the hypothalamus controls temperature regulation, some may feel hot/ cold variations too, others may experience sugar crashes because of variations in cortisol. While vagal toning is key for helping to rebalance the central nervous system, addressing any imbalance of adrenal hormones may be needed.[80] The adrenal glands may not be getting good signals from the hypothalamic control center in the brain. They may not be producing enough of the hormones needed to sustain daytime alertness.

Figure 24. SALIVARY CORTISOL AND DHEA

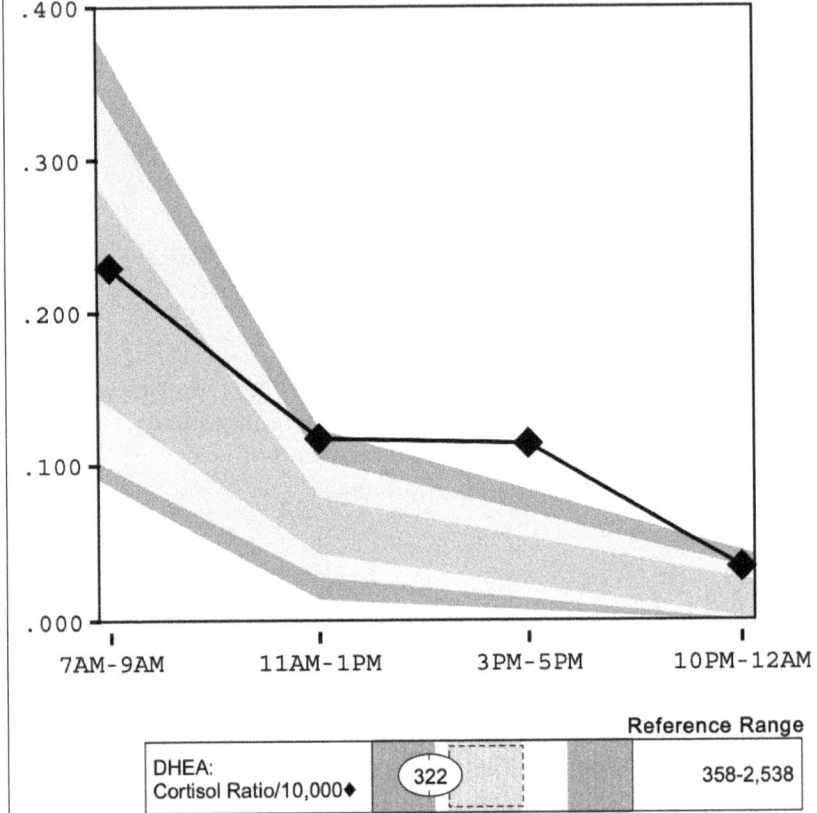

Genova 24-hour salivary testing showing adrenal dysregulation showing 4 pm cortisol peak and low morning DHEA level

Blood tests can include baseline morning cortisol, dehydroepiandrosterone (DHEA-S) levels, ACTH, and serum aldosterone. These tests are suitable for diagnosing adrenal insufficiency—a more severe and life-threatening form of adrenal failure that is fortunately uncommon. If your morning cortisol blood test shows low cortisol and low DHEA-S, you may have adrenal insufficiency. Abnormal tests are usually followed by an adrenal stimulation test, which is diagnostic. Adrenal insufficiency is treated with a low dose of physiologic steroids like Cortef/hydrocortisone, and prescription mineralocorticoids like Florinef/fludrocortisone, to mimic natural adrenal function. Many people benefit from improving their sleep quality and resetting circadian rhythms first, so steroids are a last resort in my practice. Fortunately, this more severe form of adrenal dysregulation is less common in Long COVID.

Most Long-COVID and CFS patients have a milder form of adrenal dysregulation that will not be captured by these blood tests mentioned. 24-hour salivary testing is better at capturing adrenal dysregulation. This test includes cortisol and DHEA levels measured throughout the day and is offered by many integrative physicians. DHEA and cortisol should both peak first thing in the morning, and levels drop around lunchtime. The levels continue to drop throughout the afternoon and into the evening. If either cortisol or DHEA levels are below baseline in the morning and they peak in the afternoon, this is adrenal dysfunction, and it results in a picture that looks a lot like jetlag. Figure 24 shows an example of a salivary cortisol test in a Long Hauler who reported daytime fatigue and nighttime insomnia. His morning cortisol levels were normal, but his DHEA levels were low. His cortisol peaked around 4 pm when it should have been dropping. In his case, morning DHEA supplementation and wearing amber glasses in the afternoon corrected the imbalance.

If you experience daytimes sleepiness and nocturnal insomnia, there are a few things you can do:

Blue Light Glasses in the Morning

Blue light signals your pineal gland to stop producing melatonin, a sleep hormone. Photoreceptors in the retina signal the brain it is time to be awake and produce the neurochemicals which support a wakeful state, including cortisol and epinephrine.

Amber Glasses in the Afternoon

It is helpful to reset your circadian rhythm by avoiding blue light exposure in the evening. Typically, cortisol levels fall after 1pm and continue falling throughout the day to promote easy entry into rest mode at night. Amber glasses filter out blue light, allowing cortisol and epinephrine to drop slowly. The pineal gland can secrete more melatonin in the evening, promoting return to natural circadian rhythms. Start using amber glasses around 1-2 pm when cortisol levels normally fall.[81]

Here's an example of blue light blocking amber glasses.[82]

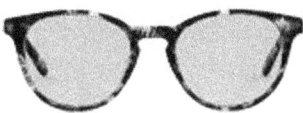

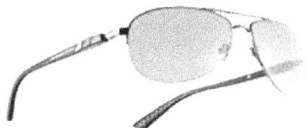

Emphasize Sleep

Your adrenals rest during sleep, therefore, it is vital that you be able to get adequate sleep. Melatonin 1-6 mg at bedtime can be helpful and it has been studied in jetlag syndrome (optimal doses unknown). You may add doxylamine, L-theanine and magnesium glycinate, or magnesium threonate at first to reset your circadian rhythm. If over-the-counter methods do not work, speak to your doctor about prescription medications to promote sleep during your recovery. You may need them temporarily to help reset your sleep/wake cycle.

Adrenal Stress End

There are a variety of supplements with herbs called adaptogens that help to decrease the adrenal stimulant drive in the evening, promoting rest and thus allowing the adrenal glands to refuel throughout the evening. Adaptogenic herbs therefore help to decrease negative impact of stress on the body. The evening blend of ashwagandha, l-theanine, magnesium and holy basil in this formula helps your adrenals reset and refuel. Too much fight-or-flight causes fatigue, promoting a feeling of "wired but tired." Turning off fight-or-flight increases energy by allowing you to conserve energy longer. Sustained stress physiology is much like having multiple tabs open in your computer throughout the day. The battery drains quickly, and the computer shuts off too soon. Turning off unnecessary programs and tabs helps the battery life last longer. Similarly, decreasing stress physiology improves fatigue by allowing conservation of energy.

De-Glycyrrhizinated (DGL) Licorice

DGL licorice in the morning helps to support adrenal function by increasing output of cortisol and helping to increase blood pressure. Licorice also has aldosterone-like effects which helps regulate salts. It is a good choice if you experience low blood pressure symptoms. Doses studied include 100-400 mg in the morning, up to 2 weeks in a row to prevent potassium imbalances. It can be safely used for longer if you have potassium checks periodically. Smaller doses of 100 mg daily are safe for daily use according to the WHO. DLG licorice is also helpful for symptoms related to gastritis and acid reflux. DGL is approved for use as an additive in foods since 1985 in the US and has the Generally Recognized as Safe (GRAS) status. However, licorice should be avoided in those with high blood pressure.[83]

If your blood levels of DHEA are low, supplement with 50 mg of DHEA in the morning to support adrenal function, then taper the dose by 10 mg every week.

It is important during your recovery to avoid re-exposure to new viral infections as much as possible to prevent renewing immune inflammation. Should you get re-exposed to COVID, the COVID protocol will support faster resolution, just add the immune support listed in figure 2 in the chart by Dr. Yanuck.

Contact to your primary care physician immediately after you have a positive COVID test to see if you are eligible for a new drug called Paxlovid. Paxlovid is the first FDA approved anti-viral medication for COVID infections and can be prescribed for those at risk for complications. There is emerging evidence that early use of Paxlovid may help decrease occurrence of COVID Long Haul.[84] At the time of this writing people at risk include older adults (aged 50 or older), those diagnosed with asthma, smokers (current or former), overweight conditions, diabetes, pregnancy, immune compromise, mental health disorders, substance use disorders, and cardiovascular disease. For updated guidelines, please check out the CDC.gov website.[85]

Summary

- Adrenal dysregulation is sometimes called "adrenal fatigue," and feels like jetlag: daytime sleepiness, difficulty falling asleep at night, difficulty regulating temperature. It is caused by dysfunction in brain regulatory centers such as the vagus and hypothalamus. The hypothalamus controls hormones and adrenal function.
- Adrenal insufficiency is a severe, life-threatening form of adrenal failure and, fortunately, it is rare. Testing for adrenal insufficiency can include morning cortisol, aldosterone, and DHEA-S levels. If abnormal, this can be followed by an adrenal stimulation test. Adrenal insufficiency testing is not sensitive enough to detect milder forms of adrenal dysregulation, which are much common in Long-COVID and CFS sufferers.
- 24-hour salivary home kits are available for cortisol and DHEA. They are much more sensitive for picking up adrenal dysregulation or "adrenal fatigue." These tests are usually prescribed by integrative physicians, but some are commercially available. Lifeextension.com offers salivary testing for purchase.
- Blue light glasses stimulate alertness in the morning.
- Amber glasses in the afternoon after 1 pm are helpful in restoring circadian rhythms and decreasing inappropriate evening cortisol peaks.
- Emphasize sleep: magnesium, melatonin, and adrenal stress end can be helpful at night.
- DGL licorice can be helpful during the day. DGL licorice can increase

blood pressure and should be avoided in hypertensives. Though 100 mg of daily licorice is deemed safe by the WHO, the higher doses are not recommended for use beyond two weeks if using 400 mg or more. If using DGL for longer, have your potassium levels monitored by a physician periodically.

- If your morning DHEA levels are low on 24-hour salivary testing, temporary DHEA supplementation can be helpful, starting at 50 mg doses each morning and tapering by 10 mg every 1-2 weeks until off.

CHAPTER 13

Viral Reactivation and Pathogen Burden

"An inefficient virus kills its host. A clever virus stays with it."
James Lovelock

C ertain viruses never leave your body, and they can be reactivated when the immune system is burdened with sustained inflammation, such as in Long COVID. Viruses such as Epstein-Barr (EBV), Herpes (HSV1-8), Cytomegalovirus (CMV) and VZV (Chickenpox and Zoster) all belong to the Herpes family and can be reactivated in the post-viral state.

HSV 1-2 is common and is estimated to affect 80-90% of the population.[86] EBV is even more common, estimated to affect 95% of the population. Most of us have been exposed to them during our lifetime and have immunity against them by forming immunoglobulin (IgG) antibodies, but they never really leave our bodies. In a healthy individual, these viruses are present in our body in such tiny amounts that they do not cause any symptoms, so long as the immune system can suppress the virus successfully. During the chronic inflammation of Long COVID, or with CFS/ME, we often see these opportunistic pathogens thrive and tests reveal increased viral titers, which contribute to inflammation. These viruses are called "opportunistic" because they take advantage of an immune system that is weakened by another infection to manifest themselves. A bit how the kids run amok when the parents are out of the house. These viruses are also called "neurotrophic" meaning "loves nerves" since they like to live near nerve endings and often end up causing inflammation of the neighboring neurons. Herpetic viruses therefore can cause symptoms of nerve inflammation like nerve pain, migraines, neuropathy, that plague many of those with CFS or Long COVID. But not always. Sometimes they just drain your energy and your brain.

Nearly all of us have IgG antibodies to EBV, so this is not a surprising finding. The presence of IgG antibodies to EBV or HSV simply means we have protective immunity. A better marker for EBV reactivation is the EBV EA or "early antigen." This test is available through Quest labs. The presence of IgM antibodies to EBV or HSV raises concern for reactivation since IgM antibodies are a response to an acute infection. Another clue is finding the IgG antibody levels to be raised three times or more above the upper limits of normal. This could reflect a higher viral burden and could be causing your symptoms of fatigue, headaches, or nerve pain.[87] We do not have as good assays for HSV or for CMV as we do for EBV, but an increasing number of studies are linking post COVID gastrointestinal inflammatory symptoms to CMV reactivation. An astute clinician might suspect CMV reactivation it in a Long Hauler with gastrointestinal symptoms. Viral PCR assays can be helpful in determining how high is the viral burden in your body.[88]

The good news is that anti-viral drugs effective against Herpes 1 and 2 are also effective against the entire family of herpesviruses, including EBV. If you benefit from a trial of an antiviral like Acyclovir, or Famciclovir, this could be an important clue to add an anti-viral regimen to the COVID protocol I have described. I recommend the amino acid lysine 3 grams daily in divided doses for any of the herpes viruses.[89] If lysine alone does not suppress the infection, it is possible to add monolaurin supplements 3 grams daily in divided for an active herpes virus infection.[90] Once the infection has cleared after two or three weeks, maintenance suppression dosing is 1 gram daily of lysine or 1 gram daily of monolaurin. I like to add immune support to help the body clear the virus quickly and this can be accomplished by adding echinacea purpurea or reishi mushrooms.

As I mentioned in the toxin chapter, if you feel worse when you start any anti-viral, you may be experiencing "die off" effects. Consider supporting liver detoxification by adding either NAC or glutathione. You may also need to ramp up the dosing more slowly over two-three weeks.

Herpes/EBV Virus Protocol
- Lysine 3 grams in divided doses for 2-3 weeks
- (optional) add Monolaurin 3 grams daily in divided doses for 2-3 weeks
- (optional) add NAC or glutathione 2 grams daily in divided doses for any die-off effects, especially in the first week.

Maintenance Dosing
- Lysine 1 gram daily, or
- Monolaurin 1 gram daily

Combine lysine supplementation with a low-arginine diet since arginine competes with lysine in the body. Nuts and seeds are rich in arginine.

An emerging theory of Long COVID is that the immune system has not fully cleared some of the COVID viral proteins, even after the infection is gone. The immune system has now learned to become highly reactive to these protein remnants, and it generates inflammation. There is emerging data that this could be true, but studies are still ongoing. If you would like to read more on this data, you can look at the LIINC studies performed at UCSF. Some patients with COVID Long Haul have had resolution or improvement in their symptoms after getting vaccinated and boosted. This could be from more effective clearance of any remaining viral particles. Others have not improved, so the verdict is not final. As of this writing, persistence of COVID viral fragments in tissue remains an emerging, though probable, theory. Because the protocol we discussed includes immune-enhancing botanicals like vitamin D and zinc, and because quercetin has direct COVID anti-viral properties, the protocol should be helpful for COVID Long Haulers who may still be clearing viral particles from their system.

Summary

- Viral reactivation with viruses in the herpes family, such as EBV and HSV, can occur in Long COVID and contribute to fatigue. These viruses are "neurotrophic" meaning they love to be near nerves. They can increase nerve inflammation and nerve pain and contribute to fatigue.
- Labs concerning for EBV reactivation include detection of EBV early antigen, EBV IgM antibodies, or an increase in EBV IgG antibodies or EBV VCA antibodies over 3 x the upper limit of normal. These tests are available at LabCorp or Quest.
- Lysine and monolaurin have anti-viral properties specific to viruses in the herpes family, including HSV and EBV. An anti-viral protocol may help your symptoms if they are caused by these viruses. With lysine, it is important to avoid high arginine foods, such as nuts and seeds, since arginine competes with lysine in the body.

CHAPTER 14

Use Of Light Therapy-Phototherapy

"Darkness cannot drive out darkness; only light can do that."
Martin Luther King, Jr

Your nose is the perfect microbial castle. Virally contaminated air enters it and finds a warm, moist environment with caverns behind the nose where it can set up residence—your sinuses. Therefore, your nose is the nidus, or "nest" for breeding upper respiratory infections, including COVID and the common cold. The sinuses are very vascular, filled with capillaries and can serve as a gateway to your bloodstream. Passage of air makes the nose the ideal gateway to your lungs. Unlike humans, who breed a few times in their life if they are lucky, microbes replicate every 30 minutes. It pays to be aggressive and proactive while the microbial burden is still small, and the symptoms are mild. Good hand and nasal hygiene immediately after indoor social or other high-risk events can be helpful. I recommend gargling with saline water or an antiseptic, plus using a sinus rinse after each high-risk event, such as an indoor gathering. Beyond that, at the first sign of a potential infection, such as sneezing, there are some tools you can use. Light therapy has been used for decades in medical and research laboratories to sterilize equipment because of its broad antimicrobial effects.

The emergence of the SARS-CoV-2 and subsequent variant strains in the Coronavirus pandemic has made it clear that new technologies to combat viral infections are needed. UV light has broad anti-microbial properties, including anti-viral, anti-bacterial, and anti-fungal properties. New technology using UV light can be a potentially useful tool.

Traditionally, UV-C is used in the laboratory settings but is toxic to humans

Figure 25. ULTRAVIOLET LIGHT AND SKIN PENETRATION

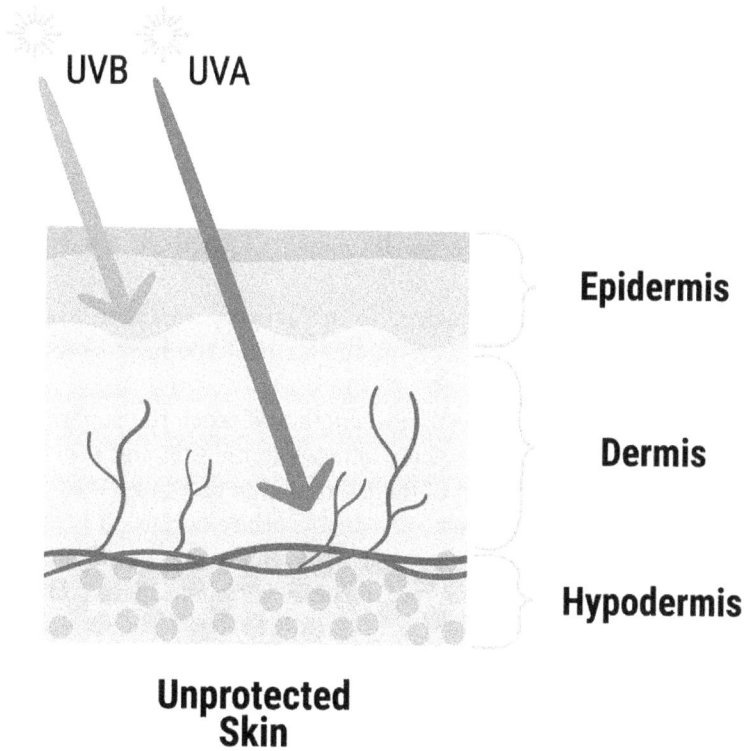

UVB   UVA

Epidermis

Dermis

Hypodermis

Unprotected Skin

[Copyright: shutterstock.com]

by inducing direct DNA damage. UV-B is also able to induce some DNA damage and is responsible for sunburns. It is used in some clinical settings in small amounts to treat diseases such as psoriasis. UV-A, however, is a long wave UV light that is safe for short-term human use. We are exposed to mostly UV-A and some UV-B when we are exposed to natural sunlight. A 2015 study found that UV-A does not affect gene expression in human cells.[91] and possesses anti-microbial properties. UV-A's longer wavelength gives it deeper penetration than other forms of UV light therapy, allowing it to sterilize sinus cavities even when applied topically. (See Figure 25.) UV-A is 95% of our normal daily skin exposure. While UV-B has been associated with skin cancer formation, long-term exposure to UV-A has been linked to wrinkle formation.

Upper respiratory viral infections begin in the nasal cavity after exposure to droplets or aerosols, and then seed into the lower respiratory tract. Early eradication of sinus infections can therefore be protective against the development of a subsequent respiratory infection. [Figure 26] In a 2020 study of patients with Coronavirus pulmonary infection, a UVA light therapy via internal wand application into the lungs was found effective.[92] Eradicating early viral infections, including coronavirus infections and Influenza, can have broad applications for population health and widespread consumer use.[93]

There are three forms of UV light: UV-A, UV-B and UV-C

- UV-A rays have a longer wavelength that can penetrate the middle layer of your skin (the dermis). UV-A rays are 95% of skin UV exposure in broad daylight and have been associated with wrinkle formation after long-term exposure.
- UV-B rays have a short wavelength that reaches the outer layer of your skin (the epidermis). They are more energetic and have been linked to skin cancers.
- UV-C rays have the shortest wavelength and reach the superficial layer of the skin. They can cause burn injuries to the skin and eyes and have the highest energy portion of the UV radiation spectrum. UV-C radiation from the sun does not reach the earth's surface because it is blocked by the ozone layer in the atmosphere. The only way that humans can be exposed to UV-C radiation is from an artificial source, like a lamp or laser.

UV radiation, in the form of lasers, lamps, or a combination of these, are sometimes used to treat patients with certain diseases who have not responded to other methods of therapy. Also known as phototherapy, this method of UV exposure is performed by a trained healthcare professional under the supervision of a dermatologist. Phototherapy can help treat unresponsive and severe cases of several diseases, including rickets, psoriasis, and eczema.

You can use UV-A light in the form of a light pen or UV light and apply to the maxillary and nasal sinus cavities to sterilize them. This is commonly called black light. Since most viral respiratory infections start at the nasal cavity, applying UV light can prevent a new infection by sterilizing this point of entry. I recommend application UV-A light after any high-risk contact, like indoor settings, flights, and at the first sign of congestion or sneezing

There are several UV-A flashlights and pen lights that are available commercially on Amazon that are safe for daily use. Because of its more open, long wave, UV-A penetrates deep enough to reach the inner cavities of the sinuses. It may just take a little longer than the more efficient UV-C. I recommend using UV-A light for 15 minutes at a time, and directing the light to each maxillary sinus cavity. If needed, UV-A light can be applied to the forehead area where the frontal sinus cavity lies. The UV lamp should have a wavelength of 390-400 nm and be used only15 minutes at a time, up to 3 times daily. When using UV lamps, remember to avoid the eye are or use

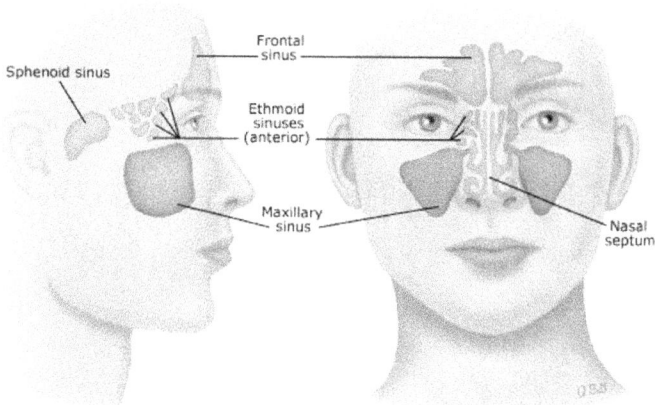

Figure 26. PARANASAL SINUS ANATOMY

Schematic drawing showing location of the frontal, ethmoid, maxillary, and sphenoid sinuses—uptodate.com/contents/image/print?imageKey=ONC%2F78790

amber protective lenses, as UV light of all frequencies can damage retinal light receptors. Most commercially available UV lamps will be in the range of 395 nm–400 nm and can be purchased for approximately 10 US dollars.

Summary

- Your nose is the entryway for upper airway infections. The warm, moist, oxygen-filled sinus cavities behind the nose can become nests for many microbes, including viruses, bacteria, and fungi.
- Good oral, nasal, and hand hygiene can be helpful prevention after any high-risk exposure. Regular handwashing, sinus rinses, gargling after indoor events are preventative.
- UV-A light has been proven safe for human use and has anti-viral properties as well. UV-A's longer wavelength can reach sinus cavities where viruses and other microbes can nest. It has been clinically tested and found effective against COVID.
- There are many low-cost commercially available UV-A pens available for purchase though online retailers. UV-A light (395 nm – 400 nm) can be applied for 15 minutes up to 3 times daily. Avoid shining UV-A light directly into the eyes.

CHAPTER 15

Preparing Your Body for the Vaccine

"Before anything else, preparation is the key to success."
Alexander Graham Bell

Most people can get vaccinations with no adverse consequences. If you are in this category and do not have any vaccine hesitancy, you can skip this chapter. Common symptoms of temporary fatigue, malaise, arm-swelling, and tenderness at the site of the injection are self-limited for most.

However, many patients I see with underlying chronic fatigue syndrome, autoimmune disorders, and those with more complex medical histories will report another story. They report more severe and prolonged consequences of vaccination, such as fatigue lasting a week or more, leading to a fear of subsequent vaccination and boosters. While current Pfizer and Moderna vaccines have created a movement of vaccine hesitancy that has been highly polarized and politicized in the United States, vaccine hesitancy is nothing new. The Moderna and Pfizer vaccines have been associated with the classical myalgias, fatigue and local injection pain that are typical of many other vaccines, though they seem to be more pronounced in some. Other more serious side effects have been reported, such as clots and myocarditis, but fortunately they have been exceedingly rare.

Most vaccine reactions are not due to what you might think. Vaccines are prepared with two components. The antigen is the component that your immune system reacts to, resulting in the production of protective antibodies. The second component is the adjuvant. It is a molecule that causes an inflammatory response, and it serves to jumpstart your immune system to respond to the antigen, instead of ignoring it. Adjuvant comes from the Latin word "adiuvare" meaning "to help" because they help the vaccine be effective. Adjuvants are thus the unsung heroes of protective immunity. They make vaccines more effective, especially in certain age groups such as babies and the elderly, where it is harder to induce a strong immune response.

However, this means that adjuvants cause the reactivity and vaccine side effects because they provoke inflammation, both locally and systemically. Modern adjuvants are based on oils such as squalene, an ingredient used as a moisturizer and present in many skin care products. It has a record of safety and is present in many vaccines, including our annual influenza vaccine. The Moderna and Pfizer m-RNA vaccines have lipid emulsion nanoparticles, and while technically they are not an adjuvants in the classical sense, they similarly elicit immune-stimulating properties, much like other oil-based adjuvants.[94] Indeed, the m-RNA by itself is not thought to create much of an immune reaction if given by itself. The immune system simply ignores it.[95]

In people who have little to no underlying inflammation, this combination works very well. The immune system wakes up enough to pay attention to the vaccine and generates protective antibodies. But for those that are already chronically inflamed, there is a higher chance of having vaccination side effects. You can slap your immune system to become awake, but what happens if you slap an immune system that is already chronically inflamed and angry?

There are reports of anaphylactoid reactions with the COVID vaccines resulting in wheezing and hives. This reaction is likely from a histaminic response to the lipid nanoparticle and is not considered a reaction to the m-RNA antigen itself. Those who have these reactions are likely already Th2 dominant and may excess histamine production in their body. The mast cell activation protocol works well here and taking an antihistamine before the vaccine can be helpful as well. For those with a history of anaphylactic shock in response to the vaccine, or other more serious reactions such as clotting, this vaccine will be contraindicated. I would like to address the more common side effects of extended malaise and fatigue in this section.

The best way to lower your risk of vaccine side effects such as prolonged malaise and fatigue is to lower your systemic inflammation prior to getting the vaccine. Starting one week before, I recommend starting a strict anti-inflammatory diet, with complete elimination of dairy, sugar, processed meats, while increasing SMASH-C fish intake and intake of cruciferous vegetables. If you have been straying from the diet, and have reincorporate cheese, yogurt, ice cream, sweets, and snacks with cured meats, this is the time to clean up your diet and fully detoxify your body.

The day before the vaccine, I recommend eating only vegetables and fatty fish as a source of protein. The day of the vaccine you may even consider intermittent fasting, which means delaying breakfast time and having an antioxidant green smoothie for lunch incorporating celery, antioxidants such as cilantro and a scoop of collagen as a source of protein with some turmeric and ginger (for the recipe please see "detox smoothie" appendix). During intermittent fasting, I recommend keeping hydrated by drinking plenty of water. Take 3 grams of omega-3 oils, vitamin D supplementation and 1-2 grams of turmeric starting 3 days before the vaccine. If you are on the Long-Haul supplement protocol, you are already taking these vitamins and following the correct diet. I followed this detox plan myself for the second Moderna shot, since the first vaccine left me with brain fog and chronic fatigue for a full week. While I had a vigorous reaction to the second vaccine, with fevers, chills and even bone pain, the malaise and fatigue were completely gone the next day.

Finally, if you have a tendency towards vaccine reactions, space out your vaccinations by three to four weeks, to allow your body to recover from one inflammatory response before challenging it again with another antigen. In this scenario, you would space your influenza vaccination and your COVID booster by three to four weeks. Consider rescheduling the vaccine if you are under the weather and potentially fighting another infection.

These recommendations do not apply to the general population and therefore they are not widely recommended by the medical community. It has helped my patients with autoimmune issues, CFS syndrome and those with vaccine hesitancy because of prior reactions. Having a plan has helped my patients regain a measure of control over their symptoms, eliminate fear, and decrease vaccine hesitancy.

Vaccine Day Smoothie
- 2 scoops of collagen protein
- 1 cup of chopped organic celery
- 1 cup of: Choice of cilantro, basil, mint, or parsley
- Choice of Lemon juice or yuzu juice
- 1 cup of organic blueberries
- 1 cup of water
- Optional: add 3 slices of ginger
- Optional: add a source of chlorophyll such as spirulina or chlorella

Summary

- Vaccine side effects are often from vaccine adjuvants, not the actual vaccine antigen. Adjuvants are usually lipid-based nanoparticles which activate the immune system, helping to make the vaccine effective. Adjuvants accomplish this by activating inflammation.
- Decreasing inflammation in your body before a vaccine can help reduce side effects.
- I recommend a strict anti-inflammatory diet the week leading up to the vaccine, and taking anti-inflammatory supplements such as turmeric, fish oil, vitamin D included in the protocol.
- Intermittent fasting and hydration can be helpful on the day of the vaccine. A smoothie filled with antioxidants the day of the vaccine is recommended.
- If you tend to have prolonged vaccine side effects, consider spacing out your vaccines by three to four weeks to allow full resolution of inflammation between vaccines.

Conclusion

L
ong COVID is a complex and debilitating condition that benefits from a systematic and multi-modal approach. The good news is that you don't have to carry this weight any longer. There is much you can do to resolve your symptoms and get your life back on track, including diet, supplements, and stress reduction at home. Because fatigue is a symptom of something gone awry in the body and it is not by itself a diagnosis, it can have multiple causes. There are many roads that lead to Rome, they say. There are many paths leading to fatigue, too. Over the years, I have created categories, or "buckets" in my brain so I could systematically address each with my patients. I have now shared them with you.

Inflammation was the first bucket we discussed, and it is a very important bucket to address. Dietary approaches include the anti-inflammatory diet, the low histamine diet, and lectin elimination. Inflammation can have many sources, which I divide into five categories: classic inflammation, histamine-mediated inflammation, gut inflammation, brain inflammation, and immune inflammation, the last three often being looped together into a triangle of gut-brain-immune dysfunction. Addressing the various sources of inflammation alone may resolve your symptoms, as it has for many of my patients. We discussed that mast cell activation is common in both CFS and Long COVID, and how a low histamine diet can be helpful if you suspect you have symptoms related to histamine excess.

While inflammation is the biggest bucket, we went over three other buckets that can cause Long-COVID symptoms: too many toxins, nutrient deficits, and high stress physiology. Although it's easier to think of these concepts as separate buckets, in the body, everything is looped together through noisy chemical crosstalk. Neuroinflammation contributes to stress, and stress physiology contributes to brain inflammation. That's one loop. Then there is the gut-brain-immune axis. That's another loop. Let's not forget the vagal-hypothalamus-adrenal axis, yet another loop. It's a bit like entering a room where individuals are having discreet conversations, but the sound that emerges is noisy chatter that can be hard to understand.

The supplement protocol in this book addresses classic inflammation, histamine-mediated inflammation, and toxins. Combined with the proper diet, this protocol can be powerful and resolve many cases of fatigue. When patients do not respond to the protocol, I notice they often have additional gastrointestinal inflammation or immune activation, through either autoimmunity or pathogen burden like EBV reactivation. In that case, addressing gut health or decreasing pathogen burden is necessary to improve brain symptoms and to improve immune function. Finally, decreasing stress physiology by prioritizing sleep, by gradual pacing of activity, and by engaging in breath work are important ways to resolve brain inflammation while improving vagal tone.

This book is by no means a comprehensive account of everything that might go wrong in the body to create Long-Haul symptoms. I have gone over the commonest and highest yield pathways I have seen in my treatment of Long-COVID patients and CFS patients. Someone wiser and more experienced than I may well have a more refined approach. Emerging evidence may inform future modifications to this protocol.

My goal in writing this book was to make the Long-COVID protocol accessible to everyone, and to empower patients with knowledge of their condition so they can start their recovery without delay. The earlier you implement the protocol, the sooner you can start your recovery. The COVID pandemic has highlighted deep inequities in our health care system, and regrettably, not everyone has access to integrative medicine specialists. Those fortunate to have access to integrative medicine may experience long wait times after the referral has been placed. Others may find integrative medicine doctors in their community to be unaffordable. By making the protocol public, I desire to open fair access to integrative healing methods for anyone who may want to explore this approach. Most interventions discussed in this book, including diet and supplements, do not require specialty consultation and can be self-directed.

In the two years since the COVID pandemic began, rapid advances in medicine created vaccines and new anti-viral drugs, multiplying our options for effective prevention and treatment. I hope that this protocol adds one more tool to your COVID toolbox, and that it embarks you on a journey of continuous healing and well-being.

In health,

Carla Kuon, MD

Acknowledgements

I am profoundly indebted to my mentor, Dr. Donald Abrams, who taught me integrative oncology and who patiently polished the initial rough drafts of this book into somewhat readable prose. My sincere thanks to Dr. Samuel Yanuck, whose functional immunology course deepened my understanding of the immune drivers of chronic illness, and whose wise lessons and clinical pearls have heavily informed my practice, this book, and the protocol. A big thank you to Danica Cowan, MS, RD, integrative dietitian, who helped me with the creation of the nutrition appendixes and whose teamwork is invaluable in my daily care of patients. Great appreciation goes to my staff. Their dedication makes my work with patients possible every day. I am most deeply grateful for my patients. They have taught me so much over the years. Because of their patience and their feedback, with some trial and error, I have been able to refine the approach which I share with you in this book. Finally, I am grateful to God for my own health journey. My struggles with chronic fatigue and brain fog resulting from an autoimmune illness planted the seeds of empathy, curiosity, and the dedication to help others who struggle with chronic illness.

APPENDIX 1

The Anti-Inflammatory Diet

Making Dietary Changes—Where to Start

Making significant dietary changes can be challenging. If all this seems daunting, it's better to start slow than not start at all. Incorporate one change per day. However, the faster you incorporate changes, the faster you will see results. Here are some tools to help you get started.

Food Journaling

Food journaling has many benefits. It promotes mindfulness, can be used as a foundation for developing your meal plan, and if working with a nutritionist provides a basis for targeted nutrition advice. Even a simple food journal can be very helpful. You can start with one-word entries—no weighing or measuring required. You can use a notebook, word processor, spreadsheet, or a food journaling app. Below are a few decent apps:

Food Journaling Apps
- Foodility. Simple free food journaling app.
- MySymptoms. Allows you to track food and symptoms and helps identify potential food sensitivities. Costs about $5, flat fee, no subscription.

Meal Planning

Planning meals ahead of time and scheduling time to cook is one of the best ways to improve the quality of our diets. Our meal planning work-sheet can help you create your own personalized meal plan. Have a backup plan, ideally multiple! You may want to batch cook and freeze some meals and/or have a reasonably healthy go-to takeout order. Depending on bud-get, you may find meal kit services or meal planning platforms to be helpful when getting started.

Anti-inflammatory Diet Basics

Pro-inflammatory Foods to Avoid

- Sugar (in all forms)
  - If you must have something sweet, choose less processed options. Sweeteners like stevia or monk fruit are acceptable substitutes.
- Refined carbohydrates (white bread, white flour products)
- Processed meats
- Highly processed "junk" food
- Dairy
  - If you must have diary, fermented dairy like kefir is preferable, and avoid cow products (goat or sheep kefir).
  - Substitute butter for clarified organic ghee (high heat cooking)
  - Substitute perilla oil for vegetable oils like canola oil (low heat cooking)

Foods to Include

- Vegetables
  - Minimum 5 servings/day, or 2 ½ cups (Serving is ½ a cup or 1 cup of raw) leafy greens
  - Focus on broccoli family/cruciferous vegetables. Broccoli sprouts are especially beneficial.
- Fruits
  - Minimum 3 servings/day (standard serving around ½ a cup) Especially berries, pomegranate
  - Ideally have half your meal fruits and vegetables, emphasis on non-starchy vegetables
- Seafood
  - 3-4 servings/week
  - Low mercury, high omega-3 seafood
- Whole grains
  - 3-5 servings/day
  - Avoid wheat, barley, rye if gluten sensitivity is a concern
  - The less processed the better (think steel cut oats as opposed to Cheerios or instant oatmeal)
- Organic non-GMO soy (unless autoimmune, soy/lectin concerns)
  - Tofu
  - Tempeh
  - Edamame
  - Avoid processed soy (think fake meat alternatives)
- Mushrooms

- · Especially shitake, maitake, other Asian mushrooms
- · Always cook your mushrooms!
- Herbs and spices
  - · Turmeric
  - · Ginger
  - · Cilantro, etc.
- Beans & legumes
  - · 1-2 servings/day
  - · Pressure cooked if lectins are a concern, avoid kidney beans

Consume in Limited Quantities
- Land Animal protein
- Grass feed beef
- Pastured chicken
- Organic, omega-3 eggs

Nutrition Recommended Reading

Nutrition Websites
- Anti-inflammatory diet:
  osher.ucsf.edu/putting-nutrition-practice-tips-making-dietary-changes
- Dr. Weil's anti-inflammatory pyramid handout:
  drweil.com/diet-nutrition/anti-inflammatory-diet-pyramid/dr-weils-
  anti-inflammatory-diet/

Cookbook Recommendations
Anti-Inflammatory diet cookbooks:
- *The Complete Ant-Inflammatory Diet for Beginners* by Dorothy Calimeris
  and Lulu Cook, RDN
  - · Simple anti-inflammatory recipes, with two-week meal plans, includ-
    ing shopping lists and background info on the anti-inflammatory diet.
- *The Power of Yum* by Rebecca Katz
  - · Flexible recipe frameworks to help adapt recipes to your dietary needs
    and preferences
- *Fast Food, Good Food* by Andrew Weil, MD
  - · Recipes based on Dr. Weil's anti-inflammatory pyramid. Most recipes
    can be adapted to be vegan, vegetarian, or gluten free.

APPENDIX 2

The Low Histamine Diet

Low Histamine Diet Basics

Foods to Avoid
- All Fermented, microbially aged foods
- Canned/cured/smoked meats
- Sausage
- Aged cheeses
- Sauerkraut and other fermented vegetables
- Alcohol

Web Resources
- mastcell360.com/low-histamine-foods-list/
- histaminintoleranz.ch/downloads/SIGHI-Leaflet_HistamineElimina-tionDiet.pdf

Making dietary changes can be difficult, but you don't have to do it alone. If you need extra assistance making dietary changes, I highly recommend finding an integrative and functionally trained Registered Dietitian Nutritionist. Here are a few websites to look for qualified professionals:

Integrative and Functional Nutrition Academy:
- ifnacademy.com/meet-the-experts/meet-our-grads/

Academy of Nutrition and Dietetics:
- www.eatright.org/find-a-nutrition-expert

APPENDIX 3

The Dirty Dozen and the Clean Fifteen

The rule of skin: It is easier to remember the dirty dozen foods when you notice these are mostly foods with thin skins that are hard to peel. For example, it is hard to peel the skin off a grape or a blueberry. These foods are more likely to carry agricultural toxins. Whenever possible, buy organic.

Clean fifteen foods can be remembered when you notice many of these foods have thick peels that we discard, like avocados and onions. (See Figure 27.)

Figure 27. CLEAN FIFTEEN and DIRTY DOZEN

Clean Fifteen (Okay to buy conventional)	Dirty Dozen (Buy organic, if possible)
1. Avocados	1. Strawberries
2. Sweet corn	2. Kale, Collards, Mustard greens
3. Pineapple	3. Spinach
4. Onions	4. Nectarines
5. Papaya	5. Apples
6. Sweet peas (frozen)	6. Grapes
7. Eggplant	7. Cherries
8. Asparagus	8. Peaches
9. Broccoli	9. Pears
10. Cabbage	10. Peppers
11. Kiwi	11. Celery
12. Cauliflower	12. Tomatoes
13. Mushrooms	
14. Honeydew	
15. Cantaloupe	

osher.ucsf.edu/putting-nutrition-practice-tips-making-dietary-changes.
Used with permission.

APPENDIX 4

SMASH + C Fish

The recommended three to four servings of fish that are low in mercury and high in omega-3 fatty acids can be remembered by the mnemonic SMASH +C:

- Salmon
- Mackerel
- Anchovies
- Sardines
- Herring
- + Cod (Black Cod)

Additional resources to check out fish quality and mercury content:

- seafood.edf.org (seafood selector)
  - See EWG seafood's mercury calculator for personalized recommendations: ewg.org/consumer-guides/ewgs-consumer-guide-seafood

TIPS:

Avoid predatory fish high in the food chain: shark, swordfish, tuna, as they will have higher mercury content.

Wild caught fish preferred whenever possible. Canned sardines are an easy way to increase fish intake. Recommended brands include Crown Prince, Kirkland brands.

APPENDIX 5

Lectin-Free Diet Basics

A Lectin-free diet is recommended for anyone suffering from an auto-immune disease, or if you have inflammatory bowel disease such as ulcerative colitis, or Crohn's colitis.

Generally, high lectin-containing foods include wheat, soy, as well as foods falling under the nightshade or legume family. Consider an elimination of the following:

Foods to Avoid
- Wheat
- Soy
- Peanuts
- lentils
- Kidney beans
- White potato
- Tomato (skins and seeds, paste ok)

Recommended Reading
The Autoimmune Solution by Dr. Amy Meyers
The Wahls Protocol by Dr. Terry Wahls

Lectin-Free Cookbooks
The Autoimmune Solution Cookbook by Amy Myers
Podcast: The Lectin-free gourmet

APPENDIX 6

Supplement Protocol for Long COVID and Mast Cell Activation

Summary of the Long-COVID Protocol

Basic Protocol
- Quercetin 1500 mg daily in divided doses
- Vitamin C 1000 mg daily in divided doses
- Zinc picolinate 30 mg twice daily
- Melatonin 3-6 mg at night (the optimal dose is unknown)
- Vitamin D3 5000 u/day–increase as needed to achieve a high normal range.
- NAC 1500-2700 mg daily in 2-3 divided doses
- Turmeric 1000-2000 mg in divided doses. Alt: Resveratrol 1000 mg daily (with fat/food)
- Omega-3 (either fish oil or vegan algae oil 3 grams daily in divided doses
- Low salt (2.3 grams) and high potassium (except for kidney impairment) anti-inflammatory diet.
- Optional: Famotidine 40mg BID (reduce dose with kidney impairment)

Basic Protocol with Added Mast Cell Stabilization
(Mast Cell Support = QBC + Perilla)
- Quercetin 1500 mg daily in divided doses (liposomal preferred)
- Bromelain 1200 units-2400 units in between meals
- Vitamin C 1000 mg in divided doses
- Perilla 150 mg twice daily (suggested Perilla brands: Pure Encapsulations or Metagenics)

- Zinc picolinate 30 mg twice daily
- Melatonin 3-6 mg at night (the optimal dose is unknown)
- Vitamin D3 5000 u/day–increase as needed to reach the upper normal levels.
- NAC 1500-2700 mg daily in 2-3 divided doses
- Omega-3 (either fish oil or vegan algae oil) 3 grams daily in divided doses
- Low salt (2.3 grams) and high potassium (except for renal impairment) anti-inflammatory diet
- Optional: Famotidine 40mg BID (reduce dose with renal impairment)

Optional for Mast Cell Activation

If you are intolerant to either quercetin of bromelain, choose 3 mast cell activators to combine with Perilla. For example, you can substitute bromelain with astragalus, rutin, or luteolin below. If levels of B2 and ferritin are low, correct those nutrients as well.

- Astragalus 1 gram twice daily
- Rutin 50 mg daily
- Luteolin 50 mg daily
- Vitamin B2 100-200 mg daily if low
- Vitamin B3 25-50 mg daily: start with 25 mg of niacin to prevent niacin flush. Alt: can use NAD+ or NMN.
- Iron Bis-glycinate 25 mg twice daily if ferritin below 100
- Consider adding Benadryl or Vistaril at bedtime to support sleep.

Tests to Consider
- Zinc/copper balance
- CRP
- ESR
- Ferritin
- B2
- B3 (if available)
- Vitamins A
- Vitamin D
- Plasma Histamine level (avoid antihistamines like Benadryl or Omeprazole, or Pepcid for 3 days before any blood test for histamine)
- Tryptase level

APPENDIX 7

Home Baking Soda Test to Improve Digestion

You need three digestive enzymes for proper digestion: stomach acid, pancreatic enzymes, and bile. Deficiencies in any of these three can cause indigestion, a sensation of food feeling "stuck" and acid reflux. If food can't pass through, it will come up. Pancreatic enzyme function can be checked with a stool pancreatic elastase test, and there is a simple home test to check for adequate stomach acid production. While there is no simple test for bile acids, you can check the other two and use a process of elimination to deduce if bile secretion is the issue.

You can try a simple home test called the "baking soda test" to see if you have enough stomach acid.

First thing in the morning, in a fasting state, mix ¼ teaspoon of baking soda into a cup of water. Drink on an empty stomach.

If you have stomach acid, the baking soda will react with your gastric acid to produce carbonation, resulting in burping within one minute. Much in the same way a carbonated drink would affect you.

This is a normal test.

If you don't burp, you probably lack stomach acid and would benefit from a digestive enzyme containing betaine HCL before each meal.

If you have a normal baking soda test but still have digestive issues, you might still have low pancreatic enzymes or low bile secretion. Consider trying a digestive enzyme with pancreatic enzymes before meals, or a digestive enzyme with bile salts in sequential order.

Causes of low gastric acid can include H. Pylori infection or the presence of antibodies against parietal cells, and age >50. You can request a stool test for H. Pylori and a blood test for gastric parietal cell antibodies. Age >50 has been associated with lower stomach acid activity.

APPENDIX 8

Vagal Toning Techniques

- Practice the 4-7-8 breath twice daily
- Inhale though your nose for four seconds
- Hold your breath for seven seconds
- Exhale slowly through your mouth over eight seconds with pursed lips.

Video (Courtesy of Dr. Andrew Weil)
- drweil.com/videos-features/videos/breathing-exercises-4-7-8-breath/

Other Resources for Vagal Toning
- www.stasis.life

Apps with Guided Meditations
- CALM app: calm.com
- INSIGHT TIMER: instighttimer.com
- HEADSPACE: headpsace.com

UCSF Osher Free Guided Imagery Meditations
- osher.ucsf.edu/guided-imagery-meditation-resources

Ear massage for Vagus Auricular Release
- youtube.com/watch?v=9uZ1rnKF5DU
  Gargling, and deep humming, such humming "hum" "om" activates vagal receptors in the larynx.

APPENDIX 9

Seven Questions for Vegans

Become an Informed Vegan!

A properly planned vegan/vegetarian diet does not need to result in nutrient deficits. Becoming aware of the nutrient gaps in a vegan/vegetarian diet, and planning meals accordingly with appropriate supplementation can prevent the metabolic deficiencies which result in chronic inflammation and chronic fatigue.

1. Do you know if you have an amino acid deficiency?

Complete proteins include all of the essential amino acids.

Lysine, tryptophan, and methionine can be low in vegan diets. These amino acids are important for energy production and neurotransmitter/mood support.

While eggs, quinoa and freekeh contain complete proteins, few other plant sources have the full range of amino acids. Consider supplementation with amino acid formulas or with Braggs Amino acids. Labs include a fasting plasma amino acid profile.

2. Do you know your B 12 status?

B12 is not found in the plant kingdom as it is produced by bacteria. B12 is important for brain function, energy, and methylation of several important functions in the body. Labs to check B12 status include fasting B12, homocysteine, and methylmalonic acid levels.

3. Do you know your iron status?

Iron is an important component of heme, a carrier for oxygen delivery throughout the body. Iron deficiency can result in cold hands and feet, exercise intolerance, excessive lactic acid production through anaerobic metabolism, and chronic fatigue. Iron is important for the Krebb's cycle, a metabolic pathway that generates energy in the body. Therefore, iron deficiency can mimic fibromyalgia symptoms. Labs to check iron status include ferritin and serum iron binding capacity. Optimal ferritin levels should be around 100 ng/ml. Levels less than 60 ng/ml are likely contributing to symptoms of fatigue. Iron deficiency can contribute to ineffective clearance of histamine in the body, resulting in elevated plasma histamine levels.

4. Do you know your omega-3 status?

Plant omega-3 sources of alpha linolenic acid (ALA) are found in walnuts, flaxseeds and hemp seeds as well as their oils. Humans only convert between 0.5% to 5% of these plant omega's into EPA and DHA. EPA and DHA are the most bioavailable omegas and important for cardiovascular and brain support. EPA and DHA are also highly effective at combating inflammation. Vegans are more susceptible to inflammatory conditions if they do not supplement with EPA/DHA. EPA/DHA can be found in fish oils; DHA-rich algae oils can be used for strict vegans.

5. Do you know if you are getting enough calcium?

Calcium is present in many non-dairy sources including leafy greens, soy, beans and broccoli. However, calcium from plant sources in not effectively absorbed due to the presence of oxalic acid found in leafy greens. Oxalic acid binds calcium and decreases its absorption. Ensure you are getting enough vitamin D3 to help you absorb calcium from dietary sources and consider calcium supplementation if needed. Labs include vitamin D, serum calcium and parathyroid hormone levels. An elevated parathyroid hormone could indicate low calcium stores.

6. Do you know your zinc status?

Zinc is an essential mineral and important in functions ranging from immune support, carbohydrate metabolism and neurotransmitter function, including dopamine production. Zinc deficiency can result in hair loss and skin rashes, as well as poor skin healing, in addition to immune deficiencies and mood disorders. Zinc competes with copper in the body so both fasting zinc and copper levels should be checked together. The ideal ratio should be approximately 1:1, and both should be near 100 ng/ml.

7. Do you know if you are getting enough iodine?

Iodine is important to support thyroid hormone production and estrogen metabolism. Iodine is present oysters, seaweed, and to a lesser degree in crustaceans. Vegetables and plants from nutrient poor soils in the US are low in iodine content. Those avoiding iodized salts and who are vegetarians are at risk for iodine deficiency. There are no serum tests for iodine deficiency, though a spot urine test level of less than 150 $\mu g/L$ is concerning for iodine deficiency.

—Adapted from Dr. Gregory Plotnikoff, M.D, co-author of "Trust Your Gut" (Conari/Red Wheel, 2013) standinguptopots.org/plotnikoff-articles

Recommended Initial Testing for Nutritional Deficiencies in Vegan/Vegetarian Diets

- Fasting B12, Methylmalonic acid, B2
- Vitamin D
- High sensitivity CRP (elevated in either vitamin D deficiency or if there is a deficiency of DHA/EPA omega-3's)
- ESR
- Homocysteine
- Fasting Zinc/copper
- Ferritin
- Plasma amino acids
- Plasma histamine and tryptase level
- Fasting B12, Methylmalonic acid, B2
- Vitamin D
- High sensitivity CRP (elevated in either vitamin D deficiency or if there is a lack of omega-3s)
- ESR
- Homocysteine
- Fasting Zinc/copperFerritin
- Plasma amino acids
- Plasma histamine and tryptase

APPENDIX 10

Protocol for Herpes Viruses (Herpes, EBV, CMV, Zoster Virus)

Herpes/EBV Virus Protocol
- Lysine 3 grams in divided doses for 2-3 weeks
- (optional) add Monolaurin 3 grams daily in divided doses for 2-3 weeks
- (optional) add NAC or glutathione 2 grams daily in divided doses for any die off effects, especially in the first week.

Maintenance Dosing
- Lysine 1 gram daily, or
- Monolaurin 1 gram daily

APPENDIX 11

Vaccine Day Detox Smoothie

Vaccine Day Smoothie
- 2 scoops of collagen protein
- 1 cup of chopped organic celery
- 1 cup of: Choice of cilantro, basil, mint or parsley
- Choice of Lemon juice or yuzu juice
- 1 cup of organic blueberries
- 1 cup of water
- 3 slices of ginger
- Optional: add scoop of spirulina or chlorella

Start your preparation seven days before the vaccine, by following a strict anti-inflammatory diet. If you are not already doing so, consider taking the anti-inflammatory supplements listed in the protocol in full doses, including vitamin D, vitamin C and fish oil omegas.

APPENDIX 12

Modified CHOP-POTS Exercise Protocol

Courtesy of Children's Hospital of Philadelphia
- Handout link: dysautonomiainternational.org/pdf/CHOP_Modified_ Dallas_POTS_Exercise_Program.pdf

The Structure of Training Calendars

There is a series of 8 training calendars that are provided for you later in this packet. Where you begin will depend on your current condition.
- Months 1-4 you should only exercise in a horizontal position, here are examples:
  · Recumbent biking
  · Rowing Ergometer
  · Swimming laps or kicking laps with a kickboard
- Month 4 you can begin to use the upright bike if it is available.
- Month 5 is when you can begin further upright training (elliptical or treadmill)

Use the calendars as a week-by-week guide. We understand that you may need to move training sessions around, but please complete all the recommended training sessions within that 7-day period. You will need to do this to move forward to the next week.

One requirement is that after Maximal Steady State' workouts you must always complete a 'Recovery' workout the next day. A 'Recovery' workout is when you do anything active but keep your heart rate below the zone prescribed. Examples of recovery workouts include:
- Slow cycling at a low level on the recumbent bike
- Using a kickboard to leisurely kick laps in the pool

- Taking a walk outdoors
- Playing in the yard
- Anything active that gets you moving continuously for the prescribed amount of time

If for some reason you miss a period of workouts (illness, injury, etc.) then you should go back in the calendar and repeat the workouts. For example:
- If you miss more than 2 cardio workouts then repeat the full week
- If you miss a week, back up and repeat 1 week
- If you miss more than 2 weeks, you should restart from the beginning of the month that you are currently in. If this is too hard then you may need to back up further. The program gets progressively more difficult.

When you take time off, you lose some of your hard-earned conditioning, so it is important to repeat workouts. You may also need to return to horizontal modes of training (i.e., recumbent bike, swimming, rowing) before moving forward in the program again.

TIPS:
- Use the equipment you have access to and can tolerate training on but starting with one horizontal mode of training is key.
- Rowing with the rowing ergometer is preferred because it mimics open water rowing. People who row in the open water tend to have the largest, strongest hearts out of all competitive athletes. Rowing is great to strengthen your heart muscle! If you are unsure how to use it ask someone to show you.
- Keep the workouts spread out throughout the week. This is more beneficial than bunching them up and then taking several days off from exercising.
- Try not to take more than 2 days off from exercising. This is KEY!!
- If you cannot complete all the sessions for that week, you need to repeat that entire week again before moving forward.

The Basics of Strength Training

The strength training sessions prescribed should take you 20-30 minutes to complete. All weight training should be done using body resistance or on seated equipment. If you are unfamiliar with strength training, you should consult with a trainer to help you use proper form and technique on each machine. It is recommended that you keep a log of your exercise. The strengthening exercises are mainly for the lower body and core, and this is intentional. Lower body muscles act as pumps when they contract (as you are walking about in daily life) to return blood to your heart. Increased muscle mass in your legs means more blood returned with each step you take.

TIPS:
- Strength training can make you sore in the beginning (especially 1-2 days after the workout).
- Some people find that they can only get to the gym three to four days a week. It is fine to do your strength training at the end of your cardio workouts instead of on separate days if you prefer. If this causes you to become symptomatic, then you should try to perform on separate days.
- Take at least a day off between strength training workouts. You need to allow your muscles at least that day to recover and to build muscle.
- We do not recommend the use of free weights until you have been able to build your strength and are able to perform with good form.
- If you have joint hypermobility then you should consult with a physical therapist prior to beginning your exercise program. The therapist can teach you how to protect your joints when you exercise.

Recommended Strength Training Exercises

If you can access a gym or fitness center then we give the general recommendation to perform 3 sets of 8-10 repetitions of the following:
- **Seated leg press**
- **Leg curl**
- **Leg extension**
- **Calf raise**
- **Chest press**
- **Seated row**

You should do as many repetitions as you can on the third set. When you can do more than 10 on the third set, then you need to increase the weight you are lifting for your next session. We also ask that you perform exercises for your belly muscles such as:
- **Back extensions**
- **Anything Pilates-based that you can do on the floor.**

If you are unable to access gym equipment then you can perform exercises using body resistance or exercise bands such as:

BRIDGES

- **Perform 3 sets of 8-10 repetitions and hold each one for 10 full seconds**
- Lay with knees bent up and hip distance apart, feet flat on the floor and hands down at your sides (Picture A).
- Try to keep your shoulders relaxed and away from your ears.
- Squeeze together gluteal (buttock) muscles and slowly lift your buttocks off the surface (Picture B)
- Do NOT arch your back! Shoulder blade area should stay on the floor and belly muscles squeezing tight (to protect your low back)
- Try to count out loud to 10 to make sure you are breathing
- *To make this harder:* Place a pillow/cushion under your feet

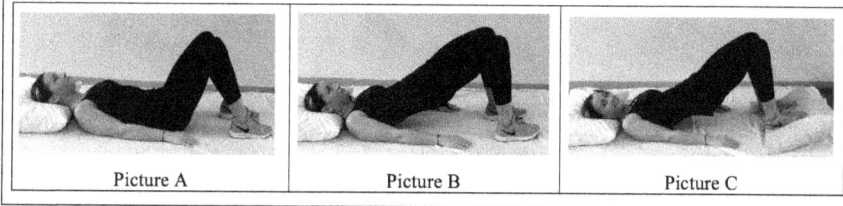

Figure 28. BRIDGES EXERCISES

Picture A   Picture B   Picture C

SEATED BALL EXERCISES

- Begin seated on an exercise ball in a safe area. Your hips and knees should be at a 90-degree angle or making an "L-shape."
- Make sure you sit up tall keeping your belly muscles engaged and your shoulders relaxed with your arms down at your sides.
- Perform 15 alternating marches while keeping your posture throughout (Picture D). **Repeat this for 3 sets of 15 alternating marches.** Then slowly kick one leg out to straighten your knee, hold 3 seconds and then begin back to start position (Picture E). **Repeat this for 3 sets of 15 alternating kicks.**
- Begin both exercises with arms down at your sides and then progress to performing with arms crossed over your chest to make it more challenging.

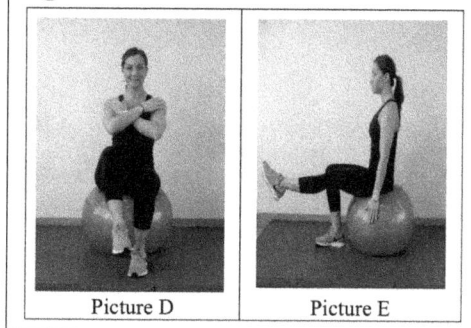

Figure 29. SEATED BALL EXERCISES

Picture D   Picture E

STRAIGHT LEG RAISES

- **Perform 3 sets of 8-10 on each leg.**
- Lay on your back with 1 knee bent and the other one straight (Picture F)
- On the straight leg: Squeeze the thigh muscle to make the knee straight. Then lift the leg up slowly until it gets near the height of the other knee. (Picture G) Hold it 1 second and then slowly lower it back down
- The goal is to keep the hips on the floor and the knee you are lifting straight
- *To make this harder:* Try it propped on your arms (Picture H) or try it with a weight strapped around your ankle

Figure 30. STRAIGHT LEG RAISES

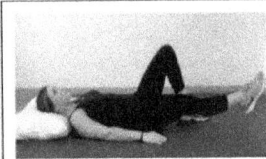
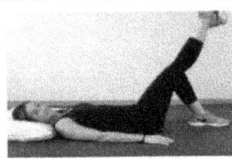
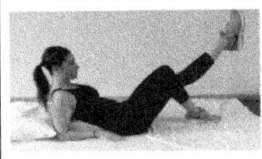

| Picture F | Picture G | Picture H |

SIDE LYING STRAIGHT LEG RAISES

- **Perform 3 sets of 8-10 repetitions**
- Lay on your side with bottom knee slightly bent and the top leg straight. The top leg should be in line with the body and not coming in front of the body (Picture I)
- Slowly lift the top leg up 8-12", hold for 1 second and then slowly lower down without turning or twisting your body (Picture J)
- *To make this harder:* Perform with an elastic band around your thighs (Picture K)

Figure 31. SIDE LAYING STRAIGHT LEG RAISES

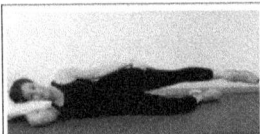
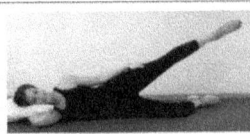
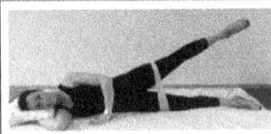

| Picture I | Picture J | Picture K |

LEG PRESSES INWARD
- **Perform 3 sets of 8-10 repetitions and hold for 5 seconds**
- Lay with knees flexed up and hip distance apart, feet flat on the floor and hands down at your sides. Place a pillow or soft ball between your thighs (Picture L)
- Squeeze your legs together into the pillow or ball- hold for 5 seconds counting out loud and then release the legs
- *To make this harder:* hold each one for 10 seconds

Figure 32: LEG PRESSES INWARD

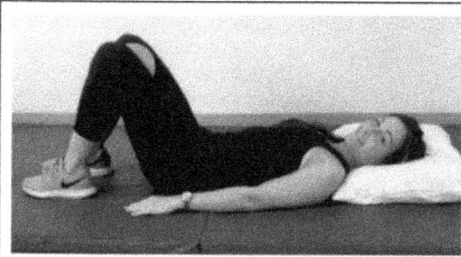

Picture L

CLAMSHELLS
- **Perform 3 sets of 8-10 repetitions on each side**
- Begin lying on either side with knees and hips bent just a little (Picture M)
- Lift the top knee off of the bottom knee, but keep your ankles together (Picture N)
- Make sure your hips and body do not twist
- *To make this harder:* try with a resistance band around your thighs

Figure 33. CLAMSHELLS

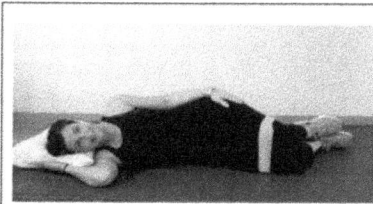

Picture M

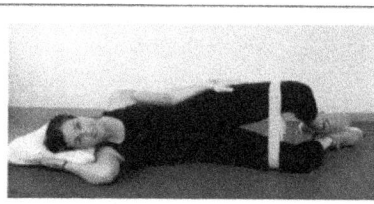

Picture N

PLANK HOLD

- **Perform 3 repetitions, holding for 15-30 seconds each time**
- Line up elbows under shoulders to start and lift your body off of the surface to make one long line (Picture O)
- Make sure you breathe while keeping your bellybutton lifted up to the ceiling and your eyes looking a few inches past your fingers to keep your head in line with your body
- *To make this harder:* Hold it longer, try 30-60 seconds

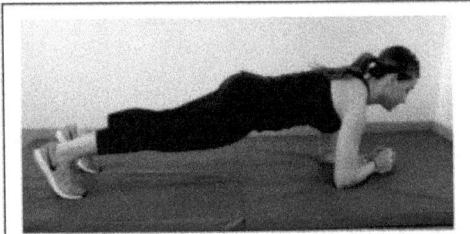

Figure 34. PLANK HOLD

Picture O

SIDE PLANK HOLD

- **Perform 3 repetitions on each side, holding for 15-30 seconds each time**
- Begin lying on your side in a long line. Feet can be stacked on top of each other or one in front of the other.
- Then line up elbow under shoulder and lift your body off of the surface to make one long line (Picture O)
- Make sure you breathe while keeping your bottom hip lifting up towards the ceiling and your head in line with your body.
- *To make this harder:* Hold it longer, try 30-60 seconds

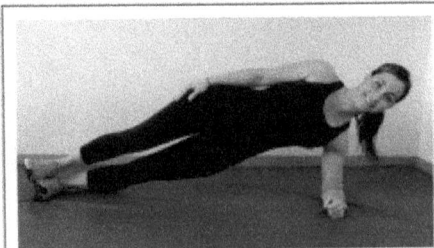

Figure 35. SIDE PLANK HOLD

Picture P

PILATES HOLD

- **Perform 8-10 repetitions on each side, holding for 10 seconds each time**
- Begin on your back with knees bent and feet on floor and arms down at your sides.
- Gently reach your hands toward your feet and bring your shoulder blades off of the floor (Picture Q)
  - Maintain slight bend in your elbows
- Try to think about keeping an apple sized object between your chin and your chest to make sure that you are not straining your neck
- Remember to breathe throughout, counting to 10

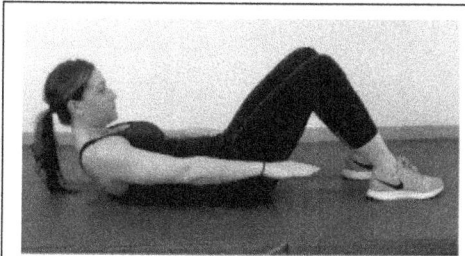

Figure 36. PILATES HOLD

Picture Q

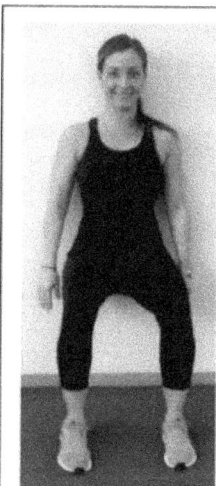

Figure 37. WALL SIT

Picture R

WALL SIT

- **Perform 3 repetitions, holding for 15-30 seconds each time**
- Lower your buttocks to knee height and then hold (Picture R)
- Make sure that feet come far enough away from wall to prevent knees crossing over
- Knees and feet should be hip distance apart and pointing straight forward
- *To make this harder:* Hold it longer, try 30-60 seconds

TIPS:
- It is okay to add new strength training exercises to your routine. You should do so slowly and know that working new muscle groups might make you sore again. If you are unsure what exercises to add you should consult with a trainer or physical therapist.
- You do not need to be able to perform all sets and reps in the first few weeks. Try to slowly build repetitions and resistance used in strengthening program over time.
- It is important to perform strength training slowly to maintain good form a prevent injuring yourself.
- If you are unsure how to perform strengthening exercises then you should consult with your physician, a trainer or a physical therapist.

The Basics of the Horizontal to Upright Cardio Training

Months 1-3 = Horizontal or Seated Training
- When beginning this exercise program you need to use equipment where you are seated or horizontal in position because upright positions will likely make your symptoms worse. Examples include:
  - Recumbent bike
  - Rowing ergometer
  - Swimming (or kicking with a kickboard)
  - Seated stepper machine

Month 4= Upright Bike
Month 5= Upright Exercise
- Elliptical (begin without arm motion and then add after a few weeks)
- Treadmill walking (no incline at first) Month 6-8 =Upright Training
- Add in use of arm motion on the elliptical and incline on the treadmill
- Make more challenging during this time as tolerated
  - Jogging and stair stepping can be tried only after you have performed either elliptical with use of arms or treadmill walking on an incline and did not have an increase in symptoms. You do not ever have to jog if you do not want to.

Warm Up and Cool Down
- Can be done on any piece of equipment and should NEVER be skipped.
- At the end of your warm up you should have your heart rate approaching

the target heart rate range for your workout.
- For the cool down, simply remove all resistance from the piece of equipment you are using and slow down.
  - In the beginning, your heart rate will take a long time to recover, but as you train more it will lower more quickly
- Try performing stretching during or after your 10 minute cool down is complete. You should hold each stretch for 30 seconds and repeat 3-4 times on each side. Only stretch to the point where you begin to feel resistance. It should feel a little uncomfortable, but it should not hurt. Here are some examples:

HAMSTRING STRETCH
- **Perform 3 sets on each leg, holding each stretch for 30 seconds**
- Sit upright with one leg long (knee straight) and the other bent in (make sure your foot does not cross underneath your leg) (Picture S). Try to keep your shoulders relaxed and away from your ears.
- Slowly and gently bend forward from the waist until you feel tension in the back of your leg or thigh. Once you feel this tension stop and hold this position for 30 seconds and repeat 3 times on each leg.
  - Do NOT round your back

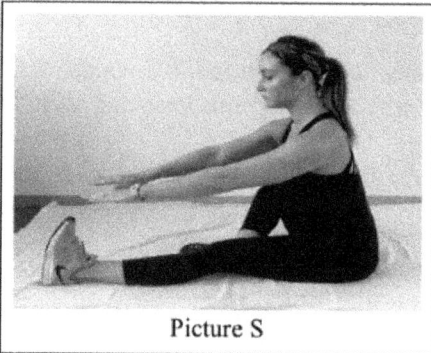

Figure 38. HAMSTRING STRETCH

Picture S

QUADRICEPS STRETCH

- **Perform 3 sets on each leg, holding each stretch for 30 seconds**
- Begin laying comfortably on your stomach. Use a long towel, sheet or dog leash to loop around your foot and gently pull until you feel tension in the front of your thigh and then hold for 30 seconds. (Picture T)
- Keep the rest of your body relaxed and do NOT let your leg rotate out to the side. Your heel should be coming straight toward your buttocks and not to the outside of it.
- You can rest your head on a pillow if you would like to decrease tension on your low back.

Figure 39. QUADRICEPS STRETCH and CALF STRETCH

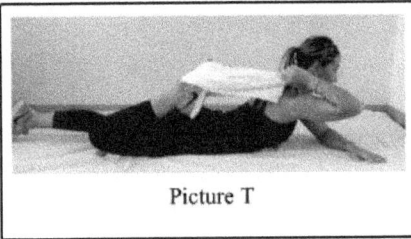

Picture T

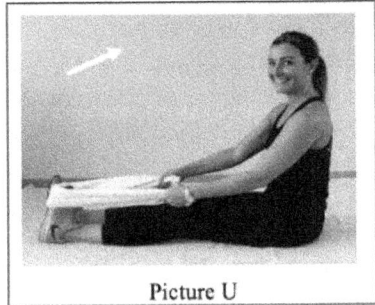

Picture U

CALF STRETCH

- Perform 3 sets on each leg, holding each stretch for 30 seconds
- Begin sitting upright with your legs stretched out long and your knee straight.
- Place a towel or sheet around the bottom of your foot and use this to gently pull your toes and foot toward you. (Picture U)
- You should feel a gentle stretch behind your lower leg and ankle. Hold this position for 30 seconds. Then repeat 3 times on each leg.

TIPS:
- This site can help you learn the rowing technique. It can be used for *any* rowing ergometer:
  - concept2.com/indoor-rowers/training/technique-videos
- If you have unbearable symptoms when first trying a more upright mode, then simply return to the horizontal or seated mode. You should then try upright exercise again a few weeks later
- If you want to use two different pieces of equipment (for example, 15

minutes on the upright bike and then 15 minutes on the rower) that is fine. Just be sure you complete the prescribed time on the training calendar with your heart rate in the appropriate training zone before cooling down.

Just be sure you complete the prescribed time on the training calendar with your heart rate in the appropriate training zone before cooling down.

Monitoring Your Heart Rate

We recommend you purchase a heart rate monitor set (a watch with a chest strap) to monitor your heart rate during cardio exercise training so you can exercise in the proper heart rate zones. These can be found online or at a large sporting goods store. You do not need to purchase an expensive model. Each cardio workout is prescribed to be within a specific heart rate range (see Training Guidelines sheet from your healthcare provider), and it is important that you complete the workout in that heart rate range. You may notice that your resting heart rate decreases with training. Or, it could be unchanged, but your heart rate response to upright posture is lower.

TIPS:
- Some monitors work even while swimming in the pool.
- If you ever question what the monitor is reading (equipment can go bad or need new batteries), simply feel your pulse at your neck or wrist and count the beats for 15 seconds and multiply by four (heart beats per minute).
- If you are unsure how to take your heart rate this guide can help you:
  - move.va.gov/download/NewHandouts/PhysicalActivity/P09_HowToTakeYourHeartRate.pdf

Endnotes

Introduction. The Rise of Pandemics

1   Larkin, HD. (2020). Global COVID-19 Death Toll May Be Triple the Reported Deaths. *JAMA*. doi.org/10.1001/jama.2022.4767
2   Vos, T. (2022). Estimated Global Proportions of Individuals With Persistent Fatigue Cognitive, and Respiratory Symptom Clusters Following COVID-19 in 2020 and 2021. *JAMA*. jamanetwork.com/journals/jama/fullarticle/2797443
3   Meng, M. (2022) COVID-19 associated EBV reactivation and effects of ganciclovir treatment. *Immunity, Inflammation and Disease*. pubmed.ncbi.nlm.nih.gov/35349757; Sacchi, M. (2021). SARS-CoV-2 infection as a trigger of autoimmune response. *National Library of Medicine*. pubmed.ncbi.nlm.nih.gov/33306235; Matyushkina, D. (2022). Autoimmune Effect of Antibodies against the SARS-CoV-2 Nucleoprotein. *Viruses*. doi.org/10.3390/v14061141; Knight, J. et al. (2021). The intersection of COVID-19 and autoimmunity. *Journal of Clinical Investigations*. jci.org/articles/view/154886

Chapter 1. Prevention

4   Howard, J. (2021). An evidence review of face masks against COVID-19. *PNAS*. doi.org/10.1073/pnas.201456411
5   Matyushkina, D. (2022). Autoimmune Effect of Antibodies against the SARS-CoV-2 Nucleoprotein. *Viruses*. doi.org/10.3390/v14061141

Chapter 2. Inflammation is One of the Key Drivers of Long-Haul Symptoms

6   Yanuck, SF. (2020). Evidence Supporting a Phased Immuno-physiological Approach to COVID-19 From Prevention Through Recovery. *Integrative Medicine, a Clinician's Journal*.

pubmed.ncbi.nlm.nih.gov/324257126

7   The WHO Rapid Evidence Appraisal for COVID-19 Therapies (REACT) Working Group. (2020). Association Between Administration of Systemic Corticosteroids and Mortality Among Critically Ill Patients With COVID-19. *JAMA*. doi.org/10.1001/jama.2020.17023

Chapter 3. The Anti-Inflammatory Diet

8   Ornish, D. (1998). Intensive lifestyle changes for reversal of coronary heart disease. *JAMA*. doi.org/10.1001/jama.280.23.2001

9   Berenson, A. B. (2013). Effect of hormonal contraceptives on vitamin B12 level and the association of the latter with bone mineral density. *Contraception*. doi.org/10.1016/j.contraception.2012.02.015

10 Weil, A. (2017). Dr. Weil's Anti-inflammatory Diet and Food Pyramid. *drweil.com*. drweil.com/wp-content/uploads/2017/06/dr-weils-anti-inflammatory-diet-and-food-pyramid-print.pdf

11 Mokhtari , R. (2017). The role of Sulforaphane in cancer chemoprevention and health benefits: a mini-review. *Cell Commun Signal*. doi.org/10.1007/s12079-017-0401-y; Zabetakis, I. (2017). COVID-19: The Inflammation Link and the Role of Nutrition in Potential Mitigation. *Nutrients*. doi.org/10.3390/nu12051466

12 Zimmermann, M. B. (2021). Global Endocrinology: Global perspectives in endocrinology: coverage of iodized salt programs and iodine status in 2020. *European Journal of Endocrinology*. doi.org/10.1530/EJE-21-0171

13 Li, R. (2016). A systematic determination of polyphenols constituents and cytotoxic ability in fruit parts of pomegranates derived from five Chinese cultivars. *Springerplus*. doi.org/10.1186/s40064-016-2639-x

14 Ianza, A. (2021). Role of the IGF-1 Axis in Overcoming Resistance in Breast Cancer. *Frontiers in Cell and Developmental Biology*. doi.org/10.3389/fcell.2021.641449

15 Wu, R. (2011). Effects of fermented Cordyceps sinensis on oxidative stress in doxorubicin treated rats. *Pharmacognosy*. doi.org/10.4103/0973-1296.165562

16 Schwenzer, H. (2021). The Novel Nucleoside Analogue ProTide NUC-7738 Overcomes Cancer Resistance Mechanisms In Vitro and in a First-In-Human Phase I Clinical Trial. *Translational Cancer Mechanisms and Therapy* doi.org/10.1158/1078-0432.CCR-21-1652

17 Balakrishnan, B. (2021). Combining the Anticancer and Immunomodulatory Effects of Astragalus and Shiitake as an Integrated Therapeutic Approach. *Translational Cancer Mechanisms and Therapy*.

doi.org/10.3390/nu13082564

18 Chunder, R. (2022). Antibody cross-reactivity between casein and myelin-associated glycoprotein results in central nervous system demyelination. *Immunology and Inflammation.* doi.org/10.1073/pnas.211703411

19 Chetty, A. (2002). Insulin-like Growth Factor-I Signaling Mechanisms, Type I Collagen and Alpha Smooth Muscle Actin in Human Fetal Lung Fibroblasts. *Pediatric Research.* doi.org/10.1203/01. pdr.0000238257.15502.f4

20 Hermanowicz, J. M. (2019). Important players in carcinogenesis as potential targets in cancer therapy: an update. *Oncotarget.* doi.org/10.18632/oncotarget.27689

21 Ianza. (2021); Pollak, M. (2008). Insulin and insulin-like growth factor signalling in neoplasia. *Nat Rev Cancer.* doi.org/10.1038/nrc2536; Wang, C. (2020). Insulin-like growth factor-I activates NFκB and NLRP3 inflammatory signalling via ROS in cancer cells. *Molecular and Cellular Probes.* doi.org/10.1016/j.mcp.2020.101583.

22 Chunder. (2022); Baspinar, B. (2020). Gluten-Free Casein-Free Diet for Autism Spectrum Disorders: Can It Be Effective in Solving Behavioural and Gastrointestinal Problems? *Eurasian Journal of Medicine.* doi.org/10.5152/eurasianjmed.2020.19230

23 Jiangin, S. (2016). Effects of milk containing only A2 beta casein versus milk containing both A1 and A2 beta casein proteins on gastrointestinal physiology, symptoms of discomfort, and cognitive behavior of people with self-reported intolerance to traditional cows' milk. *Nutrition Journal.* doi.org/10.1186/s12937-016-0147-z

24 Baune, B. (2007). Intense Sweetness Surpasses Cocaine Reward. *PLOS 1.*

Chapter 4. Histamine Inflammation, Histamine Intolerance, and Mast Cell Activation

25 Malone, R. (2021). COVID-19: Famotidine, Histamine, Mast Cells, and Mechanisms. *Frontiers in Pharmacology.* doi.org/10.3389/fphar.2021.633680

26 Weinstock, L. (2021). Mast cell activation symptoms are prevalent in Long-COVID. *International journal of infectious diseases.* doi.org/10.1016/j.ijid.2021.09.043

27 Medzhitov R. (2011). Highlights of 10 years of immunology in Nature Reviews Immunology. *Nature Reviews Immunology.*

28 Malone, R. (2021). COVID-19: Famotidine, Histamine, Mast Cells, and

Mechanisms. *Frontiers in Pharmacology.*
doi.org/10.3389/fphar.2021.633680

29 Molderings, G. (2011). Mast cell activation disease: a concise practical
guide for diagnostic workup and therapeutic options. *J Hematol Oncol*

30 Weng, Z. (2012). Quercetin is more effective than cromolyn in
blocking human mast cell cytokine release and inhibits contact
dermatitis and photosensitivity in humans. *PLOS 1;* Jarusch, R. (2014).
Impact of oral vitamin C on histamine levels and seasickness. *J Vestib
Res.*; Maintz, L. (2007). Histamine and histamine intolerance. *Am J
Clin Nutr.*

31 Imran, M. (2022). The Therapeutic and Prophylactic Potential of
Quercetin against COVID-19: An Outlook on the Clinical Studies,
Inventive Compositions, and Patent Literature. *Antioxidants.* doi.
org/10.3390/antiox11050876; Di Pierro, F. (2021). Potential Clinical
Benefits of Quercetin in the Early Stage of COVID-19: Results of a
Second, Pilot, Randomized, Controlled and Open-Label Clinical Trial.
Int J Gen Med. doi.org/10.2147/IJGM.S318949

32 Makino, T. (2003). Antiallergic effect of Perilla frutescens and its
active constituents. *Phytotherapy Research.* doi.org/10.1002/ptr.1115;
Makino, T. (2001). Effect of oral treatment of Perilla frutescens
and its constituents on type-I allergy in mice. *Biol Pharm Bull* doi.
org/10.1248/bpb.24.1206; Moon, TC. (2014). Mast cell mediators:
their differential release and the secretory pathways involved.
Frontiers in Immunology. doi.org/10.3389/fimmu.2014.00569;
Yang, S. H. (2021). Perilla Leaf Extract Attenuates Asthma Airway
Inflammation by Blocking the Syk Pathway. *Mediators Inflamm.* doi.
org/10.1155/2021/6611219; Yano, S. (2007). Dietary flavones
suppresses IgE and Th2 cytokines in OVA-immunized BALB/c
mice. *European Journal of Nutrition.* doi.org/10.1007/s00394-
007-0658-7; Yano, S. (2006). Dietary apigenin suppresses IgE and
inflammatory cytokines production in C57BL/6N mice. *European
Journal of Nutrition.* doi.org/10.1021/jf0607361; Ueda H. (2004).
Luteolin as an anti-inflammatory and anti-allergic constituent of
Perilla frutescens, *Biol Pharm Bull.* doi.org/10.1248/bpb.25.1197
2002; Takano, H. (2004). Extract of Perilla frutescens enriched
for rosmarinic acid, a polyphenolic phytochemical, inhibits
seasonal allergic rhinoconjunctivitis in humans. *Exp Biol Med.* doi.
org/10.1177/153537020422900305

33 Varilla, C. (2021). Bromelain, a Group of Pineapple Proteolytic
Complex Enzymes (Ananas comosus) and Their Possible Therapeutic
and Clinical Effects. A Summary. *Foods.* doi.org/10.3390/
foods10102249; Fathi, AN. (2022). Effect of bromelain on mast cell

numbers and degranulation in diabetic rat wound healing. *J Wound Care.* doi.org/ 10.12968/jowc.2022.31.Sup8.S4

34   Balakrishnan. (2021); Mao, S.P. (2004). Modulatory effect of Astragalus membranaceus on Th1/Th2 cytokine in patients with herpes simplex keratitis. *Chinese Journal of Integrated Traditional and Western Medicine.* PMID 15015443; Chen, S.M. (2014). Astragalus membranaceus modulates Th1/2 immune balance and activates PPARγ in a murine asthma model. *Biochem Cell Biol.* doi..org/10.1139/bcb-2014-0008; Bamodu, O. A. (2019). Astragalus polysaccharides (PG2) Enhances the M1 Polarization of Macrophages, Functional Maturation of Dendritic Cells, and T Cell-Mediated Anticancer Immune Responses in Patients with Lung Cancer. *Nutrients.* doi.org/10.3390/nu11102264

35   Casacchia, M. (1978). SAMe and histamine. *Monogr Gesamtgeb Psychiatr Psychiatry Ser.* pubmed.ncbi.nlm.nih.gov/692538

36   Maintz, L. (2007). Histamine and histamine intolerance. *Am J Clin Nutr.* doi.org/10.1093/ajcn/85.5.1185

37   Zimatkin, S. (1998). Alcohol-histamine interactions. *Alcohol and Alcoholism.* doi.org/10.1093/alcalc/34.2.141

38   Fiscella K. (2021). Transforming Health Care to Address Value and Equity: National Vital Signs to Guide Vital Reforms. *JAMA.* doi.org/10.1001/jama.2021.9938; Fiscella, K. (2000). Addressing Socioeconomic, Racial, and Ethnic Disparities in Health Care. *JAMA.* doi.org/10.1001/jama.283.19.2579; NIH Office of the Director. (2019). Populations Underrepresented in the Extramural Scientific Workforce. *National Institutes of Health.* diversity.nih.gov/about-us/population-underrepresented

39   Mahabadi, N. (2022). Riboflavin Deficiency. *National Center for Biotechnology Information* PMID: 29262062

40   Schnedl, W. (2019). Diamine oxidase supplementation improves symptoms in patients with histamine intolerance. *Food Sci Biotechnol.* doi.org/10.1007/s10068-019-00627-3

41   Maintz, L. (2007). Histamine and histamine intolerance. *Am J Clin Nutr.* doi.org/10.1093/ajcn/85.5.1185

Chapter 5. Toxin Overload

42   Faghihloo, M. (2018). Viruses as key modulators of the TGF-beta pathway; a double-edged sword involved in cancer. *Rev. Med. Virol.* doi.org/10.1002/rmv.1967; Hamidi, S.H. (2021). Role of pirfenidone in TGF-β pathways and other inflammatory pathways in acute respiratory syndrome coronavirus 2 (SARS-Cov-2) infection: a

theoretical perspective. *Pharmacol Rep.* doi.org/10.1007/s43440-021-00255-x S.H

43 Suran, M. (2022). EPA Takes Action Against Harmful "Forever Chemicals" in the US Water Supply. *JAMA.* doi.org/10.1001/jama.2022.12678

44 Gillezeau, C. (2019). The evidence of human exposure to glyphosate: a review. *Environmental Health.* doi.org/10.1186/s12940-018-0435-5

45 McCarthy, M. (2019). Circadian rhythm disruption in Myalgic Encephalomyelitis/Chronic Fatigue Syndrome: Implications for the post-acute sequelae of COVID-19. *Brain Behavior Immunity and Health.* doi.org/10.1016/j.bbih.2022.100412 2022; Montoya, J.G. (2017). Cytokine signature associated with disease severity in chronic fatigue syndrome patients. *PNAS.* doi.org/10.1073/pnas.171051911

46 Williams, J. (2002). Therapy of circadian rhythm disorders in chronic fatigue syndrome: no symptomatic improvement with melatonin or phototherapy. *Eur. J. Clin. Invest.* doi.org/10.1046/j.1365-2362.2002.01058.x; Beynon, A. (2009). Age and time of day influences on the expression of transforming growth factor-beta and phosphorylated SMAD3 in the mouse suprachiasmatic and paraventricular nuclei. *Neuroimmunomodulation;* Blundell, S. (2015). Chronic fatigue syndrome and circulating cytokines: a systematic review. *Brain Behav. Immun.* doi.org/10.1016/j.bbi.2015.07.004; Cambras, T. (2018). Circadian rhythm abnormalities and autonomic dysfunction in patients with Chronic Fatigue Syndrome/Myalgic Encephalomyelitis. *PLoS One* doi.org/10.1371/journal.pone.0198106; Kon, N. (2008). Activation of TGF-beta/activin signalling resets the circadian clock through rapid induction of Dec1 transcripts. *Nat Cell Biol.* doi.org/10.1038/ncb1806.https://doi.org/10.1371/journal.pone.0198106.

47 Ferreira-Gomes, M. (2021). SARS-CoV-2 in severe COVID-19 induces a TGF-β-dominated chronic immune response that does not target itself. *Nature Communications.* doi.org/10.1038/s41467-021-22210-3

48 Liu, R.M. (2009). Oxidative stress and glutathione in TGF-??-mediated fibrogenesis. *Free Radical Biology and Medicine.* doi.org/10.1016/j.freeradbiomed.2009.09.026

49 Ferreira-Gomes. (2021); Oronsky, B. (2021). A review of persistent post-COVID syndrome (PPCS). *Rev. Allergy Immunol.* doi.org/10.1007/s12016-021-08848-3

Chapter 6. The GI-Immune Axis

50 Carding, S. (2015). Dysbiosis of the gut microbiota in disease. *Microbial Ecology in Health and Disease.* https://doi.org/10.3402/mehd.v26.2619110.3748/wjg.v17.i6.750; Brzezińska-Blaszczyk , E. (1997). Intestinal mucosa-associated bacteria modulate rat mast cell reactivity. *Int J Immunopathol Pharmacol.* PMID: 12793960

51 Black, C. (2020). Global burden of irritable bowel syndrome: trends, predictions and risk factors. *Nature Reviews Gastroenterology and Hepatology* doi.org/10.1038/s41575-020-0286-8

Chapter 7. Supplement Protocol for Long Haul

52 Bakaloudi, D. (2022). A critical update on the role of mild and serious vitamin D deficiency prevalence and the COVID-19 epidemic in Europe. *Nutrition.* doi.org/10.1016/j.nut.2021.111441

53 Zhang, L. (2020). Potential interventions for novel coronavirus in China: A systematic review. *J Med Virol.* doi.org/10.1002/jmv.25707

54 Weng, 2012; Onal, H. (2021). Treatment of COVID-19 patients with quercetin: a prospective, single center, randomized, controlled trial. *Turkish Journal of Biology.* doi.org/10.3906/biy-2104-16; Di Pierro, F. (2021). Potential Clinical Benefits of Quercetin in the Early Stage of COVID-19: Results of a Second, Pilot, Randomized, Controlled and Open-Label Clinical Trial. *International Journal of General Medicine.* doi.org/10.2147/IJGM.S318949

55 Montoya, J.G. (2017). Cytokine signature associated with disease severity in chronic fatigue syndrome patients. *PNAS.* doi.org/10.1073/pnas.171051911

56 Price, N.L. (2012). SIRT1 is required for AMPK activation and the beneficial effects of resveratrol on mitochondrial function. *Cell Metab.* doi.org/10.1016/j.cmet.2012.04.003

57 Markus, A. (2008). Resveratrol in prevention and treatment of common clinical conditions of aging. *Clinical interventions in Aging.* PMID: 18686754; Inoue, H. (2015). Resveratrol Targets in Inflammation. *Endocrine, Metabolic & Immune Disorders—Drug Targets.* doi.org/10.2174/1871530315666150316120316; Nakata, R. (2012). Recent advances in the study on resveratrol. *Biol Pharm Bull.* doi.org/10.1248/bpb.35.273

58 Hua, J. (2007). Resveratrol inhibits pathologic retinal neovascularization in Vldlr(-/-) mice. *Invest Ophthalmol Vis Sci.* doi.org/10.1167/iovs.10-6496

Chapter 8. Nutrient Deficiencies

59 Bakaloudi, 2022; Dror, A. (2022). Pre-infection 25-hydroxyvitamin D3 levels and association with severity of COVID-19 illness. *PLoS One.* doi. org/10.1371/journal.pone.0263069
60 Veninga, K.S. (1984). Effects of oral contraceptives on vitamins B6, B12, C, and folacin. J Nurse Midwifery. doi.org/10.1016/0091-2182(84)90169-1
61 Pasricha, S. (2020). Iron deficiency Anaemia. *The Lancet.*
62 Deichmann, R. (2010). Coenzyme Q10 and Statin-Induced Mitochondrial Dysfunction. *The Oschner Journal;* Rundek, T. (2004). Atorvastatin Decreases the Coenzyme Q10 Level in the Blood of Patients at Risk for Cardiovascular Disease and Stroke. *JAMA.* doi. org/10.1001/archneur.61.6.889
63 Canavan, C. (2014). The epidemiology of irritable bowel syndrome. *Clinical Epidemiology.* doi.org/10.2147/CLEP.S40245
64 Fatima, R. (2022). Achlorhydria. *StatPearls Publishing.* PMID: 29939570; Feldman, M. (1996). Effects of aging and gastritis on gastric acid and pepsin secretion in humans: a prospective study. *Gastroenterology.* doi.org/10.1053/gast.1996.v110.pm8612992; Kawashima, J. (2010). Change in function of gastric acid secretion by aging. *Nihon Rinsho.*

Chapter 9. Neuroinflammation, Vagal Tone, and Stress Physiology

65 Acanfora, D. (2022). Impaired Vagal Activity in Long-COVID-19 Patients. *Viruses.* doi.org/10.3390/v14051035
66 Basharat, S. (2022). Vagus Nerve Stimulation for the Treatment of Post–COVID-19 Condition. *Can Health Tehnologies.*
67 Boezaart, A. (2021). Treatment of Stage 3 COVID-19 With Transcutaneous Auricular Vagus Nerve Stimulation Drastically Reduces Interleukin 6 Blood Levels: A Report on Two Cases. *Neuromodulation.* doi.org/10.1111/ner.13293
68 Cragg, G. M. (2010). Huperzia serrata PKS1 accepts bulky N-methylanthraniloyl-CoA (14) starter, and carries out three condensations with malonyl-CoA (1) to produce 1,3-dihydroxy-N-methylacridone. *Comprehensive Natural Products II.* sciencedirect.com/topics/agricultural-and-biological-sciences/huperzia-serrata; Zheng, L. F. (2011). Reduced expression of choline acetyltransferase in vagal

motoneurons and gastric motor dysfunction in a 6-OHDA rat model of Parkinson's disease. *Brain Res.* doi.org/10.1016/j.brainres

69 Gamabe, R. (2020). Cholinergic Modulation of Glial Function During Aging and Chronic Neuroinflammation. *Frontiers in Cellular Neuroscience;* Memorial Sloan Cancer Center (2022). Huperzia serrata. *MSKCC.org.* www.mskcc.org/cancer-care/integrative-medicine/herbs/huperzia-serrata

70 Liu, L. (2017). Choline ameliorates cardiovascular damage by improving vagal activity and inhibiting the inflammatory response in spontaneously hypertensive rats. *Nature Scientific Reports.* doi.org/10.1038/srep42553

71 Pavlov, V. (2008). Brain acetylcholinesterase activity controls systemic cytokine levels through the cholinergic anti-inflammatory pathway. *Brain Behav Immun.* doi.org/10.1016/j.bbi.2008.06.011

72 Szypuła, W. (2020). Huperzine A and Huperzine B Production by Prothallus Cultures of Huperzia selago (L.) Bernh. ex Schrank et Mart. *Molecules.* doi.org/10.3390/molecules25143262

73 Awogbindin, I. O. (2021). Microglial Implications in SARS-CoV-2 Infection and COVID-19: Lessons From Viral RNA Neurotropism and Possible Relevance to Parkinson's Disease. *Frontiers in Cellular Neuroscience.* doi.org/10.3389/fncel.2021.6702; Albrecht, D. (2019). Brain glial activation in fibromyalgia – A multi-site positron emission tomography investigation. *Brain, Behavior, and Immunity.* doi.org/10.1016/j.bbi.2018.09.018; Bouayed, J. (2021). The link between microglia and the severity of COVID-19: The "two-hit" hypothesis. *J Med Virol.* doi.org/10.1002/jmv.26984

74 Younger, J. (2014). The use of low-dose naltrexone (LDN) as a novel anti-inflammatory treatment for chronic pain. *Clinical Rheumatology.* doi.org/10.1007/s10067-014-2517-2

Chapter 10. Postural Autonomic Tachycardia (POTS)

75 Raj, S. (2020). Diagnosis and management of postural orthostatic tachycardia syndrome. *CMAJ.* doi.org/10.1503/cmaj.211373

76 Murray, M. (2020). Glycyrrhiza glabra (Licorice). *Textbook of Natural Medicine.* doi.org/10.1016/B978-0-323-43044-9.00085-6

77 Roberts, L.J. 2nd, (1984). Recurrent Syncope due to Mastocytosis. *Hypertension;* Roberts, L.J. 2nd, (1982). Mastocytosis without urticaria pigmentosa: a frequently unrecognized cause of recurrent syncope. *Trans Assoc Am Physicians*

Chapter 11. Exercise Intolerance

79 Smakowski, A. (2022). Graded exercise therapy for patients with chronic fatigue syndrome in secondary care—a benchmarking study. *Disabil Rehabil*

Chapter 12. Adrenal Fatigue

80 McCarthy, M.J. (2022). Circadian rhythm disruption in Myalgic Encephalomyelitis/Chronic Fatigue Syndrome: Implications for the post-acute sequelae of COVID-19. *Brain, Behaviour, & Immunity-Health*

81 Burkhart, K. (2009). Amber lenses to block blue light and improve sleep: A randomized trial. *Chronobiology International.* doi.org/10.3109/07420520903523719; Hester, L. (2021). Evening wear of blue-blocking glasses for sleep and mood disorders: a systematic review. *Chronobiol Int.* doi.org/10.1080/07420528.2021.1930029

82 amazon.com/blue-light-blocking-glasses-men-blocker/dp/ B07ZG3P352/; https://www.amazon.com/HEALTH-LISTS-Blocking-Glasses-Better/dp/B081Y4C7G9

83 Murray, 2020; Bailly, C. (2020). Glycyrrhizin: An alternative drug for the treatment of COVID-19 infection and the associated respiratory syndrome? *Pharmacol Thera.* doi.org/10.1016/j. pharmthera.2020.107618

84 Yan Xie, (2022) Nirmatrelvir and the Risk of Post-Acute Sequelae of COVID-19. *MedRxiv preprint.*

85 Centers for Diseases Control and Prevention. (2022). Outpatient Treatment Overview. *cdc.gov/coronavirus*

Chapter 13. Viral Reactivation and Pathogen Burden

86 Wald, A. (2007). Human Herpesviruses: Biology, Therapy, and Immunoprophylaxis. Persistence in the population: epidemiology, transmission. *Cambridge University Press.* ncbi.nlm.nih.gov/books/ NBK4744

87 Jacobs, E. (2018). Etiology of Chronic Disease: A Discussion on Epstein-Barr Virus. *Journal of Cancer Biology & Treatment.* doi.org/10.24966/CBT-7546/100014

88 Weber, S. (2022). CMV seropositivity is a potential novel risk factor for severe COVID-19 in non-geriatric patients. *PLoS ONE.* doi.org/10.1371/journal.pone.0268530

89 Melano, I. (2021). Effects of Basic Amino Acids and Their Derivatives on SARS-CoV-2 and Influenza-A Virus Infection. *Viruses*. doi.org/10.3390/v13071301; Stagi, L. (2022). Blocking viral infections with lysine-based polymeric nanostructures: a critical review. *Biomaterials Science*. doi.org/10.1039/D2BM00030J

90 Barker, L. (2019). The Clinical Use of Monolaurin as a Dietary Supplement: A Review of the Literature Amino Acids and Their Derivatives on SARS-CoV-2 and Influenza-A Virus Infection. *Journal of Chiropractic Medicine*. doi.org/10.1016/j.jcm.2019.02.004]

Chapter 14. Use Of Light Therapy-Phototherapy

91 Wong, D. Y. (2015). Low-Dose, Long-Wave UV Light Does Not Affect Gene Expression of Human Mesenchymal Stem Cells. *PLoS ONE*. doi.org/10.1371/journal.pone.0139307

92 Rezaie, A. (2020). Ultraviolet A light effectively reduces bacteria and viruses including coronavirus. *PLoS ONE*. doi.org/10.1371/journal.pone.0236199

93 Leite, G. (2021). Ultraviolet-A light reduces cellular cytokine release from human endotracheal cells infected with Coronavirus. *Photodiagnosis Photodyn Ther*. doi.org/10.1016/j.pdpdt.2021.102457

Chapter 15. Preparing Your Body for the Vaccine

94 Kobiyama, K. (2022). Making innate sense of mRNA vaccine adjuvanticity. *Nature Immunology*. doi.org/10.1038/s41590-022-01168-4

95 Kariko, K. (2005). Suppression of RNA recognition by Toll-like receptors: the impact of nucleoside modification and the evolutionary origin of RNA. *Immunity*. doi.org/10.1016/j.immuni.2005.06.008

References

Introduction. The Rise of Pandemics

1   Larkin, HD. (2020). Global COVID-19 Death Toll May Be Triple the Reported Deaths. *JAMA*. doi.org/10.1001/jama.2022.4767
2   Vos, T. (2022). Estimated Global Proportions of Individuals With Persistent Fatigue Cognitive, and Respiratory Symptom Clusters Following COVID-19 in 2020 and 2021. *JAMA*. jamanetwork.com/journals/jama/fullarticle/2797443
3   Figure 1: Proal, A. (2021). Long COVID or Post-acute Sequelae of COVID-19 (PASC): An Overview of Biological Factors That May Contribute to Persistent Symptoms. *Frontiers in Microbiology*. frontiersin.org/articles/10.3389/fmicb.2021.698169/full#B50; Davis et al. (2020). Characterizing Long COVID in an international cohort: 7 months of symptoms and their impact. *medRxiv*. thelancet.com/journals/eclinm/article/PIIS2589-5370(21)00299-6/fulltext
4   Meng, M. (2022) COVID-19 associated EBV reactivation and effects of ganciclovir treatment. *Immunity, Inflammation and Disease*. pubmed.ncbi.nlm.nih.gov/35349757
5   Matyushkina, D. (2022). Autoimmune Effect of Antibodies against the SARS-CoV-2 Nucleoprotein. *Viruses*; Knight, J. et al. (2021). The intersection of COVID-19 and autoimmunity. *Journal of Clinical Investigations*. jci.org/articles/view/154886
6   Sacchi, M. (2021). SARS-CoV-2 infection as a trigger of autoimmune response. *National Library of Medicine*. pubmed.ncbi.nlm.nih.gov/33306235
7   Howard, J. (2021). An evidence review of face masks against COVID-19. *PNAS*. doi.org/10.1073/pnas.201456411
8   Yanuck, SF. (2020). Evidence Supporting a Phased Immuno-physiological Approach to COVID-19 From Prevention Through Recovery. *Integrative Medicine, a Clinician's Journal*. pubmed.ncbi.nlm.nih.gov/324257126

Chapter 1. Prevention

9   Howard, J. (2021). An evidence review of face masks against COVID-19. *PNAS*. doi.org/10.1073/pnas.201456411Howard, J. (2017).

10 Knight, J. et al. (2021). The intersection of COVID-19 and autoimmunity. *Journal of Clinical Investigations*. jci.org/articles/view/154886

11 Matyushkina, D. (2021). SARS-CoV-2 infection as a trigger of autoimmune response. *Clinical and Translational Science*. doi.org/10.1111/cts.12953

Chapter 2. Inflammation is One of the Key Drivers of Long-Haul Symptoms

12 Yanuck, SF. (2020). Evidence Supporting a Phased Immuno-physiological Approach to COVID-19 From Prevention Through Recovery. *Integrative Medicine, a Clinician's Journal*. pubmed.ncbi.nlm.nih.gov/324257126

13 The WHO Rapid Evidence Appraisal for COVID-19 Therapies (REACT) Working Group F. (2020). Association Between Administration of Systemic Corticosteroids and Mortality Among Critically Ill Patients With COVID-19. *JAMA*. doi.org/10.1001/jama.2020.17023

Chapter 3. The Anti-Inflammatory Diet

14 Ornish, D. (1998). Intensive lifestyle changes for reversal of coronary heart disease. *JAMA*. doi.org/10.1001/jama.280.23.2001.

15 Berenson, A. B. (2013). Effect of hormonal contraceptives on vitamin B12 level and the association of the latter with bone mineral density. *Contraception*. doi.org/10.1016/j.contraception.2012.02.015

16 Weil, A. (2017). Dr. Weil's Anti-inflammatory Diet and Food Pyramid. *drweil.com*. drweil.com/wp-content/uploads/2017/06/dr-weils-anti-inflammatory-diet-and-food-pyramid-print.pdf

17 Mokhtari , R. (2017). The role of Sulforaphane in cancer chemoprevention and health benefits: a mini-review. *Cell Commun Signal*. doi.org/10.1007/s12079-017-0401-y

18 Ruhee, R. T. (2018). The Integrative Role of Sulforaphane in Preventing Inflammation, Oxidative Stress and Fatigue: A Review of

a Potential Protective Phytochemical. Antioxidants. *Antioxidants.* doi. org/10.3390/antiox9060521

19   Zabetakis, I. (2017). COVID-19: The Inflammation Link and the Role of Nutrition in Potential Mitigation. *Nutrients.* doi.org/10.3390/ nu12051466.

20   Zimmermann, M. B. (2021). Global Endocrinology: Global perspectives in endocrinology: coverage of iodized salt programs and iodine status in 2020. *European Journal of Endocrinology.* doi.org/ 10.1530/EJE-21-0171.

21   Ianza, A. (2021). Role of the IGF-1 Axis in Overcoming Resistance in Breast Cancer. *Frontiers in Cell and Developmental Biology.* doi.org/10.3389/fcell.2021.641449

22   Li, R. (2016). A systematic determination of polyphenols constituents and cytotoxic ability in fruit parts of pomegranates derived from five Chinese cultivars. *Springerplus.* doi.org/10.1186/s40064-016-2639-x

23   Wu, R. (2011). Effects of fermented Cordyceps sinensis on oxidative stress in doxorubicin treated rats. *Pharmacognosy.* doi.org/10.4103/0973-1296.165562

24   Schwenzer, H. (2021). The Novel Nucleoside Analogue ProTide NUC-7738 Overcomes Cancer Resistance Mechanisms In Vitro and in a First-In-Human Phase I Clinical Trial. *Translational Cancer Mechanisms and Therapy* doi.org/10.1158/1078-0432.CCR-21-1652

25   Balakrishnan, B. (2021). Combining the Anticancer and Immunomodulatory Effects of Astragalus and Shiitake as an Integrated Therapeutic Approach. *Translational Cancer Mechanisms and Therapy.* doi.org/10.3390/nu13082564

26   Chunder, R. (2022). Antibody cross-reactivity between casein and myelin-associated glycoprotein results in central nervous system demyelination. *Immunology and Inflammation.* doi.org/10.1073/pnas.211703411

27   Chetty, A. (2002). Insulin-like Growth Factor-I Signaling Mechanisms, Type I Collagen and Alpha Smooth Muscle Actin in Human Fetal Lung Fibroblasts. *Pediatric Research.* doi.org/10.1203/01.pdr.0000238257.15502.f4.

28   Hermanowicz, J. M. (2019). Important players in carcinogenesis as potential targets in cancer therapy: an update. *Oncotarget.* doi.org/10.18632/oncotarget.27689

29   Ianza, A. (2021). Role of the IGF-1 Axis in Overcoming Resistance in Breast Cancer. *Frontiers in Cell and Developmental Biology.* doi.org/10.3389/fcell.2021.641449

30   Wang, C. (2020). Insulin-like growth factor-I activates NFκB and NLRP3 inflammatory signalling via ROS in cancer cells. *Molecular and*

Cellular Probes. doi.org/10.1016/j.mcp.2020.101583.

31 Pollak, M. (2008). Insulin and insulin-like growth factor signalling in neoplasia. *Nat Rev Cancer*. doi.org/10.1038/nrc2536.

32 Jiangin, S. (2016). Effects of milk containing only A2 beta casein versus milk containing both A1 and A2 beta casein proteins on gastrointestinal physiology, symptoms of discomfort, and cognitive behavior of people with self-reported intolerance to traditional cows' milk. *Nutrition Journal*. doi.org/10.1186/s12937-016-0147-z.

33 Baspinar, B. (2020). Gluten-Free Casein-Free Diet for Autism Spectrum Disorders: Can It Be Effective in Solving Behavioural and Gastrointestinal Problems? *Eurasian Journal of Medicine*. doi.org/10.5152/eurasianjmed.2020.19230.

34 Lenoir, M. (2007). Intense Sweetness Surpasses Cocaine Reward. *PLOS One*. doi.org/10.1371/journal.pone.0000698

Chapter 4. Histamine Inflammation, Histamine Intolerance, and Mast Cell Activation

35 Weinstock, L. (2021). Mast cell activation symptoms are prevalent in Long-COVID. *International journal of infectious diseases*. doi.org/10.1016/j.ijid.2021.09.043

36 Malone, R. (2021). COVID-19: Famotidine, Histamine, Mast Cells, and Mechanisms. *Frontiers in Pharmacology*. doi.org/10.3389/fphar.2021.633680

37 Medzhitov R. (2011). Highlights of 10 years of immunology in Nature Reviews Immunology. *Nature Reviews Immunology*.

38 Molderings, G. (2011). Mast cell activation disease: a concise practical guide for diagnostic workup and therapeutic options. *J Hematol Oncol*

39 Weng, Z. (2012). Quercetin is more effective than cromolyn in blocking human mast cell cytokine release and inhibits contact dermatitis and photosensitivity in humans. *PLOS 1*.

40 Jarusch, R. (2014). Impact of oral vitamin C on histamine levels and seasickness. *J Vestib Res*.

41 Maintz, L. (2007). Histamine and histamine intolerance. *Am J Clin Nutr*.

42 Yang, S. H. (2021). Perilla Leaf Extract Attenuates Asthma Airway Inflammation by Blocking the Syk Pathway. *Mediators Inflamm*. doi.org/10.1155/2021/6611219

43 Ishihara, T. (1999). Inhibition of antigen-specific T helper type 2 responses by Perilla frutescens extract]. Aerugi. https://doi.org/10.3390/molecules24010102

44 Yuan, J. (2022). Perilla Leaf Extract (PLE) Attenuates COPD Airway Inflammation via the TLR4/Syk/PKC/NF-κB Pathway In Vivo and In Vitro. *Frontiers in Pharmacology.* doi.org/10.3389/fphar.2021.763624

45 Makino, T. (2003). Antiallergic effect of Perilla frutescens and its active constituents. *Phytotherapy Research.* doi.org/10.1002/ptr.1115

46 Makino, T. (2001). Effect of oral treatment of Perilla frutescens and its constituents on type-I allergy in mice. *Biol Pharm Bull* doi.org/10.1248/bpb.24.1206

47 Ueda H. (2004). Luteolin as an anti-inflammatory and anti-allergic constituent of Perilla frutescens, *Biol Pharm Bull.* doi.org/10.1248/bpb.25.1197 2002

48 Moon, T. (2014). Mast cell mediators: their differential release and the secretory pathways involved. *Frontiers in Immunology.* doi.org/10.3389/fimmu.2014.00569

49 Sanbongi, C. (2004). Rosmarinic acid in perilla extract inhibits allergic inflammation induced by mite allergen, in a mouse model. *Clin Exp Allergy.* doi.org/10.1111/j.1365-2222.2004.01979.x.

50 Shin, T. Y. (2000). Inhibitory effect of mast cell-mediated immediate-type allergic reactions in rats by Perilla frutescens. *Immunopharmacol Immunotoxicology.* doi.org/10.3109/08923970009026007

51 Takano, H. (2004). Extract of Perilla frutescens enriched for rosmarinic acid, a polyphenolic phytochemical, inhibits seasonal allergic rhinoconjunctivitis in humans. *Exp Biol Med.* doi.org/10.1177/153537020422900305

52 Yano, S. (2006). Dietary apigenin suppresses IgE and inflammatory cytokines production in C57BL/6N mice. *European Journal of Nutrition.* doi.org/10.1021/jf0607361

53 Yano, S. (2007). Dietary flavones suppresses IgE and Th2 cytokines in OVA-immunized BALB/c mice. *European Journal of Nutrition.* doi.org/10.1007/s00394-007-0658-7

54 Yamazaki, U. (2002). Luteolin as an anti-inflammatory and anti-allergic constituent of Perilla frutescens. *Biol Pharm.* doi.org/10.1248/bpb.25.1197

55 Varilla, C. (2021). Bromelain, a Group of Pineapple Proteolytic Complex Enzymes (Ananas comosus) and Their Possible Therapeutic and Clinical Effects. A Summary. *Foods.* doi.org/10.3390/foods10102249

56 Varilla, C. (2022). Effect of bromelain on mast cell numbers and degranulation in diabetic rat wound healing. *J Wound Care.* doi.org/10.12968/jowc.2022.31.Sup8.S4

57 Fathi, AN. (2022). Effect of bromelain on mast cell numbers and

degranulation in diabetic rat wound healing. *J Wound Care.* doi.org/10.12968/jowc.2022.31.Sup8.S4

58 Mao, S.P. (2004). Modulatory effect of Astragalus membranaceus on Th1/Th2 cytokine in patients with herpes simplex keratitis. *Chinese Journal of Integrated Traditional and Western Medicine.* PMID 15015443

59 Shih-Ming, C. (2014). Astragalus membranaceus modulates Th1/2 immune balance and activates PPARγ in a murine asthma model. *Chinese Journal of Integrated Traditional and Western Medicine.* doi.org/10.1139/bcb-2014-0008

60 Bamodu, O. A. (2019). Astragalus polysaccharides (PG2) Enhances the M1 Polarization of Macrophages, Functional Maturation of Dendritic Cells, and T Cell-Mediated Anticancer Immune Responses in Patients with Lung Cancer. *Nutrients.* doi.org/10.3390/nu11102264

61 Liang, B. (2021). Combining the Anticancer and Immunomodulatory Effects of Astragalus and Shiitake as an Integrated Therapeutic Approach. *Nutrients.* doi.org/10.3390/nu13082564

62 Imran, M. (2022). The Therapeutic and Prophylactic Potential of Quercetin against COVID-19: An Outlook on the Clinical Studies, Inventive Compositions, and Patent Literature. *Antioxidants.* doi.org/ 10.3390/antiox11050876

63 Di Pierro, F. (2021). Potential Clinical Benefits of Quercetin in the Early Stage of COVID-19: Results of a Second, Pilot, Randomized, Controlled and Open-Label Clinical Trial. *International Journal of General Medicine.* doi.org/10.2147/IJGM.S318949

64 Weng, Z. (2012). Quercetin is more effective than cromolyn in blocking human mast cell cytokine release and inhibits contact dermatitis and photosensitivity in humans. *PLOS One.* doi.org/10.1371/journal.pone.0033805

65 Maintz, L. (2007). Histamine and histamine intolerance. *Am J Clin Nutr.* doi.org/10.1093/ajcn/85.5.1185

66 Jarisch, R. (2014). Impact of oral vitamin C on histamine levels and seasickness. *J Vestib Res.* doi.org/10.3233/VES-140509

67 Zimatkin, S. (1998). Alcohol-histamine interactions. *Alcohol and Alcoholism.* doi.org/10.1093/alcalc/34.2.141

68 Casacchia, M. (1978). SAMe and histamine. *Monogr Gesamtgeb Psychiatr Psychiatry Ser.* pubmed.ncbi.nlm.nih.gov/692538

69 NIH Office of the Director. (2022). Populations Underrepresented in the Extramural Scientific Workforce. *National Institutes of Health.* diversity.nih.gov/about-us/population-underrepresented

70 Fiscella, K. (2000). Addressing Socioeconomic, Racial, and Ethnic Disparities in Health Care. *JAMA.* doi.org/10.1001/jama.283.19.2579

71 Mahabadi, N. (2022). Riboflavin Deficiency. *National Center for*

Biotechnology Information PMID: 29262062

72 Schnedl, W. (2019). Diamine oxidase supplementation improves symptoms in patients with histamine intolerance. *Food Sci Biotechnol.* doi.org/10.1007/s10068-019-00627-3

73 Afrin, L. B. (2021). Diagnosis of mast cell activation syndrome: a global "consensus-2". *Diagnosis.* doi.org/10.1515/dx-2020-0005

Chapter 5. Toxin Overload

74 Mirzaei, H. (2018). Viruses as key modulators of the TGF-β pathway; a double-edged sword involved in cancer. *Rev Med Virol.* doi.org/10.1002/rmv.1967.

75 Hamidi, S. H. (2021). Role of pirfenidone in TGF-β pathways and other inflammatory pathways in acute respiratory syndrome coronavirus 2 (SARS-Cov-2) infection: a theoretical perspective. *Pharmacol Rep.* doi.org/10.1007/s43440-021-00255-x

76 Faghihloo, M. (2018). Viruses as key modulators of the TGF-beta pathway; a double-edged sword involved in cancer. *Rev. Med. Virol.* doi.org/10.1002/rmv.1967

77 Gillezeau, C. (2019). The evidence of human exposure to glyphosate: a review. *Environmental Health.* doi.org/10.1186/s12940-018-0435-5

78 Suran, M. (2022). EPA Takes Action Against Harmful "Forever Chemicals" in the US Water Supply. *JAMA.* doi.org/10.1001/jama.2022.12678

79 Liu, R. M. (2009). Oxidative stress and glutathione in TGF-β-mediated fibrogenesis. *Free Radic Biol Med.* doi.org/10.1016/j.freeradbiomed.2009.09.026.

80 Liu, R. M. (2009). Oxidative stress and glutathione in TGF-??-mediated fibrogenesis. *Free Radical Biology and Medicine.* doi.org/10.1016/j.freeradbiomed.2009.09.026

81 Gomes, M. F. (2021). SARS-CoV-2 in severe COVID-19 induces a TGF-β- dominated chronic immune response that does not target itself. *Nat Commun.* doi.org/10.1038/s41467-021-22210-3

82 McCarthy, M. (2019). Circadian rhythm disruption in Myalgic Encephalomyelitis/Chronic Fatigue Syndrome: Implications for the post-acute sequelae of COVID-19. *Brain Behavior Immunity and Health.* doi.org/10.1016/j.bbih.2022.100412

83 Montoya, J. G. (2017). Cytokine signature associated with disease severity in chronic fatigue syndrome patients. *PNAS.* doi.org/10.1073/pnas.171051911

84 Williams, J. (2002). Therapy of circadian rhythm disorders in chronic

fatigue syndrome: no symptomatic improvement with melatonin or phototherapy. *Eur. J. Clin. Invest.* doi.org/10.1046/j.1365-2362.2002.01058.x

85 Cambras, T. (2018). Circadian rhythm abnormalities and autonomic dysfunction in patients with Chronic Fatigue Syndrome/Myalgic Encephalomyelitis. *PLoS One.* doi.org/10.1371/journal.pone.0198106

86 Beynon, A. (2009). Age and time of day influences on the expression of transforming growth factor-beta and phosphorylated SMAD3 in the mouse suprachiasmatic and paraventricular nuclei. *Neuroimmunomodulation.*

87 Williams, J. (2002). Therapy of circadian rhythm disorders in chronic fatigue syndrome: no symptomatic improvement with melatonin or phototherapy. *Eur. J. Clin. Invest.* doi.org/10.1046/j.1365-2362.2002.01058.x

88 Beynon, A. (2009). Age and time of day influences on the expression of transforming growth factor-beta and phosphorylated SMAD3 in the mouse suprachiasmatic and paraventricular nuclei. *Neuroimmunomodulation*

89 Kon, N. (2008). Activation of TGF-beta/activin signalling resets the circadian clock through rapid induction of Dec1 transcripts. *Nat Cell Biol.* doi.org/10.1038/ncb1806.https://doi.org/10.1371/journal.pone.0198106

90 Ferreira-Gomes, M. (2021). SARS-CoV-2 in severe COVID-19 induces a TGF-β-dominated chronic immune response that does not target itself. *Nature Communications.* doi.org/10.1038/s41467-021-22210-3

91 Bludnell, S. (2015). Chronic fatigue syndrome and circulating cytokines: A systematic review. *Review Brain Behav Immun.* doi.org/10.1016/j.bbi.2015.07.004.

92 Oronsky, B. (2021). A review of persistent post-COVID syndrome (PPCS). *Clinical Review Allergy Immunology.* doi.org/10.1007/s12016-021-08848-3

Chapter 6. The GI-Immune Axis

93 Carding, S. (2015). Dysbiosis of the gut microbiota in disease. *Microbial Ecology in Health and Disease.* doi.org/10.3402/mehd.v26.2619110.3748/wjg.v17.i6.750

94 Brzezińska-Blaszczyk , E. (1997). Intestinal mucosa-associated bacteria modulate rat mast cell reactivity. *Int J Immunopathol Pharmacol.* PMID: 12793960

95 Black, C. (2020). Global burden of irritable bowel syndrome: trends,

predictions and risk factors. *Nature Reviews Gastroenterology and Hepatology* doi.org/10.1038/s41575-020-0286-8

96 Oksaharju, A. (2011). Probiotic Lactobacillus rhamnosus downregulates FCER1 and HRH4 expression in human mast cells. *World J Gastroenterol.* doi.org/10.3748/wjg.v17.i6.750

97 Medzhitov, R. (2011). Highlights of 10 years of immunology in Nature Reviews Immunology. *Nature Reviews Immunology.* doi.org/10.1038/nri3063

Chapter 7. Supplement Protocol for Long Haul

98 Dror, A. A. (2022). Pre-infection 25-hydroxyvitamin D3 levels and association with severity of COVID-19 illness. *Nature Reviews Immunology. Europe. Nutrition.* doi.org/10.1371/journal.pone.0263069

99 Zhang, L. (2020). Potential interventions for novel coronavirus in China: A systematic review. *J Med Virol.* doi.org/10.1002/jmv.25707

100 Weng, Z. (2012). Quercetin is more effective than cromolyn in blocking human mast cell cytokine release and inhibits contact dermatitis and photosensitivity in humans. *PLOS One.* doi.org/10.1371/journal.pone.0033805

101 Onal, H. (2021). Treatment of COVID-19 patients with quercetin: a prospective, single center, randomized, controlled trial. *Turkish Journal of Biology.* doi.org/10.3906/biy-2104-16.

102 Di Pierro, F. (2021). Potential Clinical Benefits of Quercetin in the Early Stage of COVID-19: Results of a Second, Pilot, Randomized, Controlled and Open-Label Clinical Trial. *International Journal of General Medicine.* doi.org/10.2147/IJGM.S318949

103 Montoya, J. G. (2017). Cytokine signature associated with disease severity in chronic fatigue syndrome patients. *PNAS.* doi.org/10.1073/pnas.171051911

104 Markus, A. (2008). Resveratrol in prevention and treatment of common clinical conditions of aging. *Clinical interventions in Aging.* PMID: 18686754

105 Hiroyasu, I. (2015). Metabolic & Immune Disorders—Drug Targets ISSN (Print): 1871-5303 ISSN (Online): 2212-3873 Resveratrol Targets in Inflammation. *Endocrine, Metabolic & Immune Disorders—Drug Targets.* doi.org/10.2174/1871530315666150316120316

106 Takahashi, N. R. (2012). Recent advances in the study on resveratrol. *Biol Pharm Bull.* doi.org/10.1248/bpb.35.273. PMID: 22382311

107 Hua, J. (2007). Resveratrol inhibits pathologic retinal neovascularization in Vldlr(-/-) mice. *Invest Ophthalmol Vis Sci.*

doi.org/10.1167/iovs.10-6496
108 China: A systematic review. *Invest Ophthalmol Vis Sci.*
    doi.org/10.1002/jmv.25707
109 Price, N.L. (2012). SIRT1 is required for AMPK activation and the
    beneficial effects of resveratrol on mitochondrial function. *Cell Metab.*
    doi.org/10.1016/j.cmet.2012.04.003

Chapter 8. Nutrient Deficiencies

110 Bakaloudi, D. (2022). A critical update on the role of mild and serious
    vitamin D deficiency prevalence and the COVID-19 epidemic in
    Europe. *Nutrition.* doi.org/10.1016/j.nut.2021.111441
111 Plotnikoff, G. (2012) Nutritional assessment in vegetarians and
    vegans: questions clinicians should ask. *Minn Med.* pubmed.ncbi.nlm.
    nih.gov/23346724
112 Dror, A. (2022). Pre-infection 25-hydroxyvitamin D3 levels and
    association with severity of COVID-19 illness. *PLoS One.* doi.
    org/10.1371/journal.pone.0263069
113 Veninga, K.S. (1984). Effects of oral contraceptives on vitamins
    B6, B12, C, and folacin. J Nurse Midwifery. doi.org/10.1016/0091-
    2182(84)90169-1.
114 Sant-Rayn, P. (2020). Iron deficiency anaemia. *The Lancet.*
    doi.org/10.1016/S0140-6736(15)60865-0
115 Canavan, C. (2014). The epidemiology of irritable bowel syndrome.
    Clinical Epidemiology. doi.org/10.2147/CLEP.S40245
116 Fatima, R. (2022). Achlorhydria. *StatPearls Publishing.* PMID:
    29939570
117 Feldman, M. (1996). Effects of aging and gastritis on gastric acid and
    pepsin secretion in humans: a prospective study. *Gastroenterology.*
    doi.org/10.1053/gast.1996.v110.pm8612992
118 Rundek, T. (2004). Atorvastatin Decreases the Coenzyme Q10 Level
    in the Blood of Patients at Risk for Cardiovascular Disease and Stroke.
    JAMA. doi.org/10.1001/archneur.61.6.889
119 Sakurada, Y. K. (2010). Change in function of gastric acid secretion by
    aging. Nihon Rinsho. https://doi.org/PMID: 21061523

Chapter 9. Neuroinflammation, Vagal Tone, and Stress Physiology

120 Acanfora, D. (2022). Impaired Vagal Activity in Long-COVID-19 Patients. *Viruses*. doi.org/10.3390/v14051035

121 Acanfora, D. & Bahsarat, S. (2022). Vagus Nerve Stimulation for the Treatment of Post–COVID-19 Condition. *Canadian Journal of Health Technologies*. doi.org/10.51731/cjht.2022.452

122 Boezaart, A. (2021). Treatment of Stage 3 COVID-19 With Transcutaneous Auricular Vagus Nerve Stimulation Drastically Reduces Interleukin 6 Blood Levels: A Report on Two Cases. *Neuromodulation*. doi.org/10.1111/ner.13293

123 Younger, J. (2014). The use of low-dose naltrexone (LDN) as a novel anti-inflammatory treatment for chronic pain. *Clinical Rheumatology*. doi.org/10.1007/s10067-014-2517-2

124 Albrecht, D. (2019). Brain glial activation in fibromyalgia – A multi-site positron emission tomography investigation. *Brain, Behavior, and Immunity*. doi.org/10.1016/j.bbi.2018.09.018

125 Gamage, R. (2020). Cholinergic Modulation of Glial Function During Aging and Chronic Neuroinflammation. *Frontiers in Cellular Neuroscience*. doi.org/10.3389/fncel.2020.577912

126 Awogbindin, I. O. (2021). Microglial Implications in SARS-CoV-2 Infection and COVID-19: Lessons From Viral RNA Neurotropism and Possible Relevance to Parkinson's Disease. *Frontiers in Cellular Neuroscience*. doi.org/10.3389/fncel.2021.6702

127 Bouayed, J. (2021). The link between microglia and the severity of COVID-19: The "two-hit" hypothesis. *J Med Virol*. doi.org/10.1002/jmv.26984

128 Zheng, L. F. (2011). Reduced expression of choline acetyltransferase in vagal motoneurons and gastric motor dysfunction in a 6-OHDA rat model of Parkinson's disease. *Brain Res*. doi.org/10.1016/j.brainres

129 Cragg, G. M. (2010). Huperzia serrata PKS1 accepts bulky N-methylanthraniloyl-CoA (14) starter, and carries out three condensations with malonyl-CoA (1) to produce 1,3-dihydroxy-N-methylacridone. *Comprehensive Natural Products II*. sciencedirect.com/topics/agricultural-and-biological-sciences/huperzia-serrata

130 Liu, L. (2017). Choline ameliorates cardiovascular damage by improving vagal activity and inhibiting the inflammatory response in spontaneously hypertensive rats. *Nature Scientific Reports*. doi.org/10.1038/srep42553

131 Pavlov, V. (2008). Brain acetylcholinesterase activity controls systemic

cytokine levels through the cholinergic anti-inflammatory pathway. *Brain Behav Immun.* doi.org/10.1016/j.bbi.2008.06.011

132 Boezaart, A. (2021). Treatment of Stage 3 COVID-19 With Transcutaneous Auricular Vagus Nerve Stimulation Drastically Reduces Interleukin 6 Blood Levels: A Report on Two Cases. *Neuromodulation.* doi.org/10.1111/ner.13293Memorial Sloan Cancer Center (2022). Huperzia serrata. *MSKCC.org.* www.mskcc.org/cancer-care/integrative-medicine/herbs/huperzia-serrata

133 Szypuła, W. (2020). Huperzine A and Huperzine B Production by Prothallus Cultures of Huperzia selago (L.) Bernh. ex Schrank et Mart. *Molecules.* doi.org/10.3390/molecules25143262

134 Younger, J. (2014). The use of low-dose naltrexone (LDN) as a novel anti-inflammatory treatment for chronic pain. *Clinical Rheumatology.* doi.org/10.1007/s10067-014-2517-2

135 Center for Disease Control and Prevention. (2022). Coronavirus Outpatient Treatment Overview. *cdc.gov.* https://www.cdc.gov/coronavirus/2019-ncov/hcp/clinical-care/outpatient-treatment-overview.html

Chapter 10. Postural Autonomic Tachycardia (POTS)

136 Raj, S. (2020). Diagnosis and management of postural orthostatic tachycardia syndrome. *CMAJ.* doi.org/10.1503/cmaj.211373

137 Murray, M. T. (2020). Glycyrrhiza glabra (Licorice). *Textbook of Natural Medicine.* doi.org/10.1016/B978-0-323-43044-9.00085-6

138 Roberts L.J. 2nd. (1984). Recurrent syncope due to systemic mastocytosis. *Hypertension.* PMID: 6202635

Chapter 11. Exercise Intolerance

139 Kincaid, B. (2011). Forever young: SIRT3 a shield against mitochondrial meltdown, aging, and neurodegeneration. *Front Aging Neurosci.* doi.org/10.3389/fnagi.2013.00048

140 Smakowski, A. (2019). Graded exercise therapy for patients with chronic fatigue syndrome in secondary care - a benchmarking study. *Front Aging Neurosci.* doi.org/10.1080/09638288.2021.1949049.

141 CHOP Modified Dallas POTS Program. *Dysautonomiainternation.org.* dysautonomiainternational.org/pdf/CHOP_Modified_Dallas_POTS_Exercise_Program.pdf

Chapter 12. Adrenal Fatigue

142 McCarthy, M. (2021). Circadian rhythm disruption in Myalgic Encephalomyelitis/Chronic Fatigue Syndrome: Implications for the post-acute sequelae of COVID-19. Brain Behavior Immunity and Health. https://doi.org/10.1016/j.bbih.2021.100347

Chapter 13. Viral Reactivation and Pathogen Burden

143 Hester, L. (2021). Evening wear of blue-blocking glasses for sleep and mood disorders: a systematic review. *Chronobiol Int.* doi.org/10.1080/07420528.2021.1930029

144 Burkhart, K. (2009). Amber lenses to block blue light and improve sleep: A randomized trial. *Chronobiology International.* doi.org/10.3109/07420520903523719

145 Murray, M. (2020). Glycyrrhiza glabra (Licorice). *Textbook of Natural Medicine.* doi.org/10.1016/B978-0-323-43044-9.00085-6

146 Yan, X. (2022). Nirmatrelvir and the Risk of Post-Acute Sequelae of COVID-19. *MedXRV preprint.* medrxiv.org

147 Bailly, C. (2020). Glycyrrhizin: An alternative drug for the treatment of COVID-19 infection and the associated respiratory syndrome? *Pharmacol Thera.* doi.org/10.1016/j.pharmthera.2020.107618

148 Wald, A. (2007). Human Herpesviruses: Biology, Therapy, and Immunoprophylaxis. Persistence in the population: epidemiology, transmission. *Cambridge University Press.* ncbi.nlm.nih.gov/books/NBK47447

149 Melano, I. (2021). Effects of Basic Amino Acids and Their Derivatives on SARS-CoV-2 and Influenza-A Virus Infection. *Viruses.* doi.org/10.3390/v13071301

150 Barker, L. (2019). The Clinical Use of Monolaurin as a Dietary Supplement: A Review of the Literature Amino Acids and Their Derivatives on SARS-CoV-2 and Influenza-A Virus Infection. *Journal of Chiropractic Medicine.* doi.org/10.1016/j.jcm.2019.02.004

151 Jacobs, E. (2018). Etiology of Chronic Disease: A Discussion on Epstein-Barr Virus. *Journal of Cancer Biology & Treatment.* doi.org/10.24966/CBT-7546/100014

152 Weber, S. (2022). CMV seropositivity is a potential novel risk factor for severe COVID-19 in non-geriatric patients. *PLoS ONE.* doi.org/10.1371/journal.pone.0268530

153 Stagi, L. (2022). Blocking viral infections with lysine-based polymeric nanostructures: a critical review. *Biomaterials Science.*

doi.org/10.1039/D2BM00030J

154 Barker, L. (2019). The Clinical Use of Monolaurin as a Dietary Supplement: A Review of the Literature Amino Acids and Their Derivatives on SARS-CoV-2 and Influenza-A Virus Infection. *Journal of Chiropractic Medicine.* doi.org/10.1016/j.jcm.2019.02.004

Chapter 14. Use Of Light Therapy-Phototherapy

155 Wong, D. Y. (2015). Low-Dose, Long-Wave UV Light Does Not Affect Gene Expression of Human Mesenchymal Stem Cells. *PLoS ONE.* doi.org/10.1371/journal.pone.0139307

156 Rezaie, A. (2020). Ultraviolet A light effectively reduces bacteria and viruses including coronavirus. *PLoS ONE.* doi.org/10.1371/journal.pone.0236199

157 Rezaie, A. (2021). Endotracheal Application of Ultraviolet A Light in Critically Ill Patients with Severe Acute Respiratory Syndrome Coronavirus 2: A First-in-Human Study. *Adv Ther.* doi.org/10.1007/s12325-021-01830-7

158 Leite, G. (2021). Ultraviolet-A light reduces cellular cytokine release from human endotracheal cells infected with Coronavirus. *Photodiagnosis Photodyn Ther.* doi.org/10.1016/j.pdpdt.2021.102457

Chapter 15. Preparing Your Body for the Vaccine

159 Kobiyama, K. (2022). Making innate sense of mRNA vaccine adjuvanticity. *Nature Immunology.* doi.org/10.1038/s41590-022-01168-4

160 Kariko, K. (2005). Suppression of RNA recognition by Toll-like receptors: the impact of nucleoside modification and the evolutionary origin of RNA. *Immunity.* doi.org/10.1016/j.immuni.2005.06.008

Appendices

161 COVID Data Tracker. Centers for Disease Control and Prevention. (2021). covid.cdc.gov/covid-data-tracker/#datatracker-home

162 WHO Coronavirus (COVID-19) Dashboard. World Health Organization. (2021). covid19.who.int/

163 Rubin R. (2020). As Their Numbers Grow, COVID-19 "Long Haulers" Stump Experts. *JAMA.* doi.org/10.1001/jama.2020.17709

164 Logue, J.K. (2021) Sequelae in Adults at 6 Months after COVID-19 Infection. *JAMA Network Open.* doi.org/10.1001/jamanetworkopen.2021.0830

165 Post-COVID Conditions: Information for Healthcare Providers. Centers for Disease Control and Prevention. (2021). cdc.gov/coronavirus/2019-ncov/hcp/clinical-care/post-covid-conditions.html

166 Nalbandian A. (2021). Post-acute COVID-19 syndrome. *Nature Medicine* doi.org/10.1038/s41591-021-01283-z

167 Collins, F. (2021). NIH launches new inititative to study "Long COVID" *National Institutes of Health.* nih.gov/about-nih/who-we-are/hin-director/statements/nih-launches-new-initiative-study-long-covid

168 Beyer, Bergman Announce Introduction Of Bipartisan COVID-19 Long Haulers Act. (2021). beyer.house.gov/news/documentsingle.aspx?DocumentID=5115

About the Author

Carla Kuon, MD is associate professor of the Department of Hospital Medicine at the University of California, San Francisco, where she created and directs the adult inpatient bone marrow transplant massage service. She is dual board certified in internal medicine and addiction medicine. She is faculty at the Osher Center for Integrative Health in San Francisco where she provides consultations in integrative oncology and integrative medicine, and she is chair of their educational case conference series. She teaches the "Food as Medicine" series for residents and students at the university. She has published works in Mayo Clinic Proceedings: Innovations, and Quality & Outcomes, and Global Advances in Health and Medicine. This is her first book.

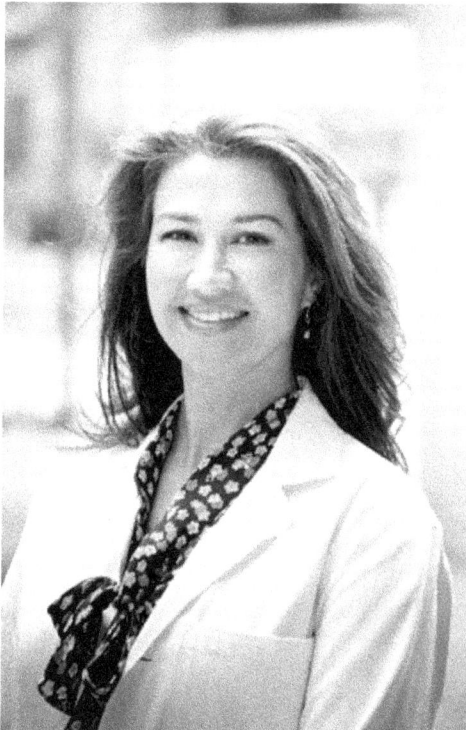

www.ingramcontent.com/pod-product-compliance
Lightning Source LLC
Chambersburg PA
CBHW032056040426
42335CB00036B/375